"We all know we're supposed to tell [...] real beauty of this book is that it understands that self-acceptance is a big fat deal and hard as hell. Luckily we now have Kate Harding and Marianne Kirby to talk us through the tough parts, with all the insight and humor of a smart, satisfying conversation."

—Wendy McClure, author of *I'm Not the New Me*

"These body-smart lessons should be common sense—but Kate, Marianne, and company deliver them with an uncommonly refreshing attitude. What a pleasure to hear these loud, proud voices from the fat-o-sphere." **—Wendy Shanker, author of *The Fat Girl's Guide to Life***

"I agree with Kate and Marianne wholeheartedly that finding the joy and freedom of good health and exercise is not the privilege of the thin, but rather the right of all of us blessed with a body. Plus-size readers and their friends and family would do well to read this positive and uplifting book." **—Megan Garcia, author and founder of *Megayoga***

"Harding and Kirby are just what the doctor ordered—well, not fat-phobic doctors, but the better kind who really care about your health and well-being. I found this book, which focuses mainly on better lives for larger women, to be helpful for big men, too. I can't think of another book out there like it!" **—Bill Fabrey, founder of the National Association to Advance Fat Acceptance**

"Two of the savviest bloggers in the fat-o-sphere now bring their fat-acceptance message to the page, with the same irreverent, hip, transgressive attitude that first turned them into online celebrities. Get ready to rethink everything you thought you knew about being fat—and, in the process, to be entertained, enlightened, impressed, and maybe even improved." **—Robin Marantz Henig, author of *Pandora's Baby* and *How a Woman Ages***

LESSONS
from the
FAT-O-SPHERE

{ Quit Dieting
and Declare a Truce
with Your Body }

KATE HARDING
and
MARIANNE KIRBY

A PERIGEE BOOK

A PERIGEE BOOK
Published by the Penguin Group
Penguin Group (USA) Inc.
375 Hudson Street, New York, New York 10014, USA
Penguin Group (Canada), 90 Eglinton Avenue East, Suite 700, Toronto, Ontario M4P 2Y3, Canada
(a division of Pearson Penguin Canada Inc.)
Penguin Books Ltd., 80 Strand, London WC2R 0RL, England
Penguin Group Ireland, 25 St. Stephen's Green, Dublin 2, Ireland (a division of Penguin Books Ltd.)
Penguin Group (Australia), 250 Camberwell Road, Camberwell, Victoria 3124, Australia
(a division of Pearson Australia Group Pty. Ltd.)
Penguin Books India Pvt. Ltd., 11 Community Centre, Panchsheel Park, New Delhi—110 017, India
Penguin Group (NZ), 67 Apollo Drive, Rosedale, North Shore 0632, New Zealand
(a division of Pearson New Zealand Ltd.)
Penguin Books (South Africa) (Pty.) Ltd., 24 Sturdee Avenue, Rosebank, Johannesburg 2196,
South Africa

Penguin Books Ltd., Registered Offices: 80 Strand, London WC2R 0RL, England

While the author has made every effort to provide accurate telephone numbers and Internet addresses
at the time of publication, neither the publisher nor the author assumes any responsibility for errors, or
for changes that occur after publication. Further, the publisher does not have any control over and does
not assume any responsibility for author or third-party websites or their content.

First edition: May 2009

Library of Congress Cataloging-in-Publication Data

Harding, Kate, 1975–
    Lessons from the fat-o-sphere : quit dieting and declare a truce with your body / Kate Harding and
Marianne Kirby.
        p.   cm.
    Includes bibliographical references and index.
    ISBN 978-0-399-53497-3
    1. Self-care, Health.   2. Physical fitness.   3. Mind and body.   I. Kirby, Marianne, 1977–
II. Title.
    RA776.95H37 2009
    613—dc22   2008054653

PRINTED IN THE UNITED STATES OF AMERICA

10   9   8   7   6   5   4   3   2   1

CONTENTS

Introduction   ix

PART ONE: HEALTH

1. ACCEPT THAT DIETS DON'T WORK   3
2. PRACTICE HEALTH AT EVERY SIZE, INCLUDING YOURS   13
3. FIND A FORM OF EXERCISE YOU LOVE   19
4. PRACTICE INTUITIVE EATING   27

PART TWO: MENTAL HEALTH

5. IF YOU THINK YOU MIGHT BE SUFFERING   43
   FROM DEPRESSION, GET HELP
6. FIND BODY-POSITIVE DOCTORS AND GO TO THEM   49
   "Fat Hatred Kills," by Barbara Benesch-Granberg   *58*
7. DON'T OBSESS IF YOU MISS A DAY AT THE GYM   64
8. DON'T WEIGH YOURSELF   70

PART THREE: SOCIALIZING

9. FIND A GOOD PARTNER   77

10. **STOP JUDGING OTHER WOMEN**   87

   "Fatness and Uplift: Not an Essay About Push-Up   *92*
   Bras," by Julia Starkey

11. **GET A HOBBY THAT HAS NOTHING TO DO WITH**   98
   YOUR WEIGHT (AND DO IT WITH OTHER PEOPLE)

12. **DON'T BELIEVE THAT ONLY SICK FREAKS WOULD WANT**   102
   TO DATE FAT WOMEN

PART FOUR: AVOIDING NEGATIVITY

13. **DON'T HANG AROUND WITH PEOPLE WHO SAY NEGATIVE**   111
   THINGS ABOUT YOUR BODY

14. **DON'T HANG AROUND WITH PEOPLE WHO SAY NEGATIVE**   118
   THINGS ABOUT THEIR OWN BODIES

15. **DON'T PARTICIPATE IN DIET TALK**   122

16. **SEEK OUT IMAGES OF HAPPY, HEALTHY, HOT, FAT WOMEN**   127

PART FIVE: GETTING DRESSED

17. **MAKE FRIENDS WITH A TAILOR/LEARN TO SEW**   135

   "'I Can't Drive in This Jacket!': And Other Reasons   *141*
   to Blame the Fit Model," by Joy Nash

18. **BUY FABULOUS CLOTHES AND WEAR THEM**   144

   "Thrift Tips for Fatties," by Cynara Geissler   *147*

19. **DON'T SHOP AT STORES THAT DON'T CARRY YOUR SIZE**   154
   (EVEN IF YOU ARE WITH THIN FRIENDS)—AND TELL
   THEM YOU'RE NOT SHOPPING THERE

20. DON'T KEEP CLOTHES THAT DON'T FIT   158

  "Depression Pants: On Buying Things Too Small as a   *162*
  Motivational Tactic," by Lesley Kinzel

PART SIX: THE MEDIA

21. TRAIN YOURSELF TO READ MEDIA REPORTS ON FAT   167
    AND DIETING WITH A CRITICAL EYE

22. READ UP ON FAT ACCEPTANCE AND   179
    THE SCIENCE OF FAT

23. QUIT WATCHING SO MUCH TV   185

PART SEVEN: GETTING YOUR HEAD ON STRAIGHT

24. GET OVER YOURSELF! THEY REALLY, REALLY AREN'T   193
    ALL LOOKING AT YOU!

  "The Wages of Visibility," by Lesley Kinzel   *198*

25. DEFEND YOUR OWN HONOR AS VIGOROUSLY   202
    AS YOU WOULD A FRIEND'S

26. ACCEPT THAT SOME DAYS WILL BE BETTER   207
    THAN OTHERS

27. DON'T PUT THINGS OFF UNTIL YOU'RE THIN!   213

CONCLUSION: DON'T DIET ANYWAY. THEY STILL DON'T WORK.   222

KATE'S ACKNOWLEDGMENTS   225
MARIANNE'S ACKNOWLEDGMENTS   227

APPENDIX I: BODY-POSITIVE RESOURCES AT THE LIBRARY   229

APPENDIX II: BODY-POSITIVE RESOURCES ONLINE   231

APPENDIX III: PLUS-SIZE CLOTHING STORES   233

ENDNOTES   235

INDEX   239

Did you ever notice that the very same magazines that tell you each and every month how to lose weight, burn more calories, fight the flab!—not to mention how to do your own smoky eye makeup, fix your hair like a celebrity, and engage in complicated pubic hair topiary—will turn right around and tell you to love your body? And then, adding insult to injury, tell you that confidence is the sexiest thing in the world?

And did you ever just want to light every one of those magazines on fire?

We're right there with you.

How on earth are you supposed to love your body when you're constantly told it's too fat, too hairy, too wrinkly, too zitty, too musky, too short, too tall, too boyish, too curvy, too sweaty, too unhealthy, too mortal, too human?

Oh, sure, there are people who claim they'll show you how. You are a goddess, they'll tell you. Light some candles and take a bubble bath and meditate on your inner womanly light. Which is just swell, if phrases like "inner womanly light" don't make you dry heave; not so for us.

Even better are the Daily Affirmation folks: Look in the mirror and say one nice thing about your body! Give yourself a hug! What the hell? Isn't the problem here that you don't like your body? Do you usually go around complimenting and hugging people you don't even like?

Learning to love your body is a long, slow process—and we mean a *long, slow* process. You can't just call a truce with your body out of nowhere; you need to engage in some hard-core peace talks first. And there's gonna be resistance. Intellectually, you might realize that everything in this book makes a lot of sense, and you really should quit hating your body posthaste. But emotionally, you'll still be so accustomed to those negative feelings about your appearance, you'll have no idea how to let go of them right away. Believe us, we know how that feels. In Chapter 22, we'll talk about the books that made us realize it was possible to be fat, healthy, and happy simultaneously, and we fervently hope this book will do the same for you. But we both had long, slow journeys (did we mention the *long* and *slow* part?) between reading those books and truly coming to like our bodies the way they are.

Chances are, you and your body have been at odds for a long time. You don't just end a decades-long feud by saying, "Well, that was silly. Let's drop it now!" (Not even if it *was* silly, which hating your body really is.) When you're used to your body being The Enemy—the stubborn foe that stands in the way of you being your best (that is, thin) self—it's really hard to start thinking kindly about it. *Really* hard.

So, to be brutally honest, we're not even going to try to tell you how to love your body. For now, we're only going tell you how to achieve détente with your body. We're just going to get you as far as a cease-fire. The good news is, in this culture, that's actually pretty freakin' far.

YEAH, I CALLED YOU FAT

Both of your devoted authors here are fat. Yeah, we said it: FAT. We can't stand the word *overweight*, because of the implication that there is a single, objectively correct weight for every human body. There ain't. The body mass index (BMI), the measure used to file people into categories of "underweight," "normal," "overweight," and "obese," is limited in its usefulness, to put it mildly. Based only on a ratio of height to weight, it doesn't take into account a host of other important factors, like age, gender, frame size, and muscle tone. And although we know some fine fatties who, because they just can't bring themselves to use the F word, would describe themselves as "Big, Beautiful Women" (BBWs) or "people of size" or indeed as "overweight," we are not those fatties. We are fat, just as we are both fairly short, both have curly hair (Marianne much more than Kate), and both wear glasses some of the time. As far as we're concerned, the word *fat* has no more moral value than those other descriptions; it just is what it is.

Of course, we're well aware that in many people's minds, *fat* not only means "having an above-average amount of adipose tissue," but a whole ton of other things that actually have nothing to do with said tissue. *Fat* can stand in for any or all of the following adjectives: disgusting, lazy, ignorant, smelly, unattractive, unhealthy, undisciplined, gluttonous, rude, sedentary, stupid. It's no wonder so many fat people themselves avoid it, or that children are taught to believe calling someone "fat" is cruel; it *is* cruel, if you mean it as an insult loaded with all of those other connotations. But fortunately or unfortunately, *fat* is also the single most efficient description of bodies that aren't, you know, thin—and we are nothing if not word nerds. We prize simplicity and accuracy. We eschew ambiguous euphemisms. We will fucking cut anyone who calls us "fluffy."

Kate, at 5'2" and about two hundred pounds, and wearing a size 16 or 18, is clinically "obese," madly in love with Lane Bryant's Right Fit jeans, and the founder of Kate Harding's Shapely Prose, one of the most popular fat acceptance blogs on the Internet (kateharding.net). And yet, she is frequently accused of not being fat *enough* to speak for fat people. *Le* sigh. Bringing the fatty-fat cred (and a whole lot more) then is Marianne, aka "The Rotund" (therotund.com), standing 5'4" on her tippy toes, weighing about 315 pounds, and rockin' size 28 or 30. Kate grew up as the thinnest kid in a fat family; Marianne (an adoptee) as the fat kid in a thin family. Between them, they can barely count how many diets they've been on, and they've lost enough weight to make up a whole other person. A whole other fat person. But, like virtually everyone who undertakes a weight-loss program (and yes, that includes "permanent lifestyle changes"—we'll get to that later), they always gained it back.

Eventually, though, we both did something even less typical than losing lots of weight on a commercial diet program and keeping it off: We gave up dieting and learned to love our fat bodies. We learned to enjoy several different kinds of exercise—walking, yoga, swimming, belly dancing, waterobics, cycling—because they were fun and made us feel better mentally and physically, as opposed to serving as a painful, dreadful punishment for fatness along with a big scoop of self-loathing. We learned to eat intuitively, which we'll tell you lots more about in Chapter 4. We learned to stop seeing disgusting, lazy, ignorant, smelly, unattractive, unhealthy, undisciplined, gluttonous, rude, sedentary, stupid women every time we looked in the mirror, and instead to see ourselves as what we really were: fat.

Just fat. Not morally bankrupt. Not pathetic. Not unlovable. Just freakin' fat—and vertically challenged and curly-haired and intermittently bespectacled, and, if we do say so ourselves, pretty damn cute. Our bodies did not mean our deaths would be attended only by a dozen cats. Our bodies did not mean we didn't deserve top-notch, respectful health care. Our bodies did not mean we were incompetent employees. Our bodies did not mean anything. They just were.

Fatness absolutely does not need to stand in the way of us living our lives with joy, pride, brio, and plenty of healthy self-respect. Unfortunately, we live in a culture that often insists it must. As our friend Melissa McEwan of the blog Shakesville (shakesville.com) puts it:

> It remains a radical act to be fat and happy in America, especially if you're a woman (for whom "jolly" fatness isn't an option). If you're fat, you're not only meant to be unhappy, but deeply ashamed of yourself, projecting at all times an apologetic nature, indicative of your everlasting remorse for having wrought your monstrous self upon the world. You are certainly not meant to be bold, or assertive, or confident—and should you manage to overcome the constant drumbeat of messages that you are ugly and unsexy and have earned equally society's disdain and your own self-hatred, should you forget your place and walk into the world one day with your head held high, you are to be reminded by the cowcalls and contemptuous looks of perfect strangers that you are not supposed to have self-esteem; you don't deserve it. Being publicly fat and happy is hard; being publicly, shamelessly, unshakably fat and happy is an act of both will and bravery.

In the following chapters, we'll encourage you to rethink the relationship between fat and health, question media reports on THE OBESITY CRISIS BOOGA BOOGA BOOGA, find a form of exercise you love, listen to what your body tells you to eat, stop listening to those conflicted women's magazines, read up on the body acceptance movement, find fabulous clothes that you can wear now instead of ten pounds from now, tell your mother to put a sock in it, and finally, once and for all, accept that diets don't cause permanent weight loss. What we're offering here is essentially a guide to all the baby steps we took on our own long, slow journeys toward being "publicly, shamelessly, unshakably fat and happy." The will and bravery to get there are up to you, dear reader. But we can tell you about some tricks that might just come in handy.

PART ONE

{ **Health** }

CHAPTER ONE

Accept That Diets Don't Work

Diets don't work. If this is news to you, hang in there with us—we've got the science to back it up. But before we hit you with the academic stuff, we want to explain why jumping off the diet bandwagon is so important to accepting your body in the first place.

Marianne and Kate both run their blogs as anti-weight-loss zones. This means there is no talking about how you just lost forty pounds on the latest diet or even how you only want to lose a few pounds for your "health." It means no diet talk, period. In the early days of our blogs, this was a really controversial position to take. A lot of dieters felt alienated by the no-diet-talk rule. But we both realized what a difference it made when we and our readers weren't being constantly bombarded with crap about how great dieting was.

Because dieting is *not* great. It's a roller coaster you climb on because you don't like your body. If you are engaging in an activity predicated on the idea that you shouldn't like your body, then body acceptance is, frankly, a goal beyond your reach for as long as you are on that ride. If you are actively seeking to change how your body looks, because it doesn't match up to an arbitrary (not to mention impossible to achieve—more on that later) beauty standard, you can't concentrate on actively changing how you view your body.

Now, we aren't discouraging dieters from learning about fat acceptance. Sometimes that disconnect between dieting and body acceptance takes a while to sort out. But do understand, right up front, that we are never going to congratulate you for starting a new weight-loss diet. We propose a different route to self-improvement, and that's what we're going to show you how to do.

By now, it's common to see headlines proclaiming that diets don't work (and the conclusions to those articles that say we should diet anyway). Even Weight Watchers started running ads that dissed dieting (because, of course, they claim Weight Watchers is not a diet) in 2008. Lots of people are hip to the diets-not-working thing in theory—but because almost no one is prepared to believe there's no safe, proven method for losing weight permanently, they'll rationalize that whatever they're doing is not a diet. What they're doing will totally work! This rationalization gives rise to the "Diets don't work, but . . ." chorus, which goes a little something like this:

Diets don't work, but . . .

- XYZ Commercial Weight-Loss Program, which is somehow not a diet, works.

- "lifestyle changes," which are somehow not diets, work.

- restricting calories for the rest of your life, which is somehow not a diet, works.

- cutting out carbs, which is somehow not a diet, works.

- eating only whole foods, which is somehow not a diet, works.

- reducing fat intake, which is somehow not a diet, works.

- "portion control," which is somehow not a diet, works.

- eating right and exercising, which is somehow not a diet (and clearly not something anyone's ever thought of before), works.

Gosh, there's so much conflicting information here! However to synthesize it? Do you suppose there's, like, a single element common to all those statements?

Ooh! Ooh! We see it! Diets don't work!

The thing that causes so much confusion (to put it charitably) is that diets do work, actually—in the short term. All diets, from cabbage soup to Weight Watchers, will cause people to lose weight. At first. But after five years, all diets have the same result: The vast majority of people who lost weight at first gained it back.

This is what people mean when they say, "Diets don't work," without adding a "but . . ." *Diets do not lead to permanent weight loss for the vast majority of people.* A slightly more efficient way of saying that is, "Diets don't work." But boy, people come out in droves to argue that one.

If you've ever looked at a commercial weight-loss program's literature, you've seen the phrase "Results Not Typical" under every picture of a triumphant former fatty showing off her new self. Let us translate that for you: "Hi! To indemnify ourselves against the world's largest class action suit, we want to make sure you're aware that our product does not work for most people! Now look back up at that picture! Don't you want to look like her? Buy our product!"

It's easy to ignore that pesky little point about the product not working, because hey, you're not typical, either! You've got the resolve! You'll be the one in the ad. Fun fact: Kate has been asked by the staff of one diet program if they could send her before and after photos to Corporate to see about making her the one in the ads on two separate occasions, years apart. She actually wasn't typical! Except . . . Two different befores, two different afters. We'll leave you to sort out what happened in between. Let's just say it was "typical."

As anyone who knew Kate between 1995 and 2002ish can attest, she was once insufferable with her endless proselytizing about "lifestyle changes." If she'd been more Internet-savvy at the time, she would have been polluting every conceivable message board with her endless rambling about how easy it is, really, once you get used to it—once you've made that lifestyle change! About how much better it feels to be thin! About how she'd taken control of her eating, her life, her destiny! About how she was never, ever, ever going back!

And boy, would she feel like an asshole now. Specifically, a fat asshole.

Here's a big secret, which we have absolutely no scientific evidence to support but would nevertheless bet every cent we have and our respective firstborns on: At least 95 percent of people who insist that "lifestyle changes" work (and who are not themselves in the business of selling weight-loss products) are fewer than five years out from the beginning of a "lifestyle change." Better known, as they will see by the end of those five years, as a "diet."

Diets do not lead to permanent weight loss for the vast majority of people. Not even if you refuse to call them diets. If your "lifestyle change" involves putting restrictions on your food intake, you will almost certainly gain back any weight you lose, and very possibly more.

SAYS WHO?

Pretty much every study that follows up with dieters five years down the line results in this conclusion. That's why most studies don't. When you read an article about how a new weight-loss trial found that some noteworthy percentage of people kept off some noteworthy percentage of weight over time, the first thing you need to ask is, "How long was the study?" You will probably find that participants were followed for two and a half years or less; often, only for one year. The next thing you need to ask is how much weight the participants in question kept off. Usually, the answer will be between 5 and 10 percent of their starting weight.

Now, let's put these numbers in perspective: Kate has twice lost more than 20 percent of her body weight—once more than 35 percent—hence the buzz from the diet center about putting her in advertisements. Both times, after one year, she'd kept nearly all of it off. After two and a half years, she'd regained some but was still maintaining well over a 10 percent loss. If researchers had been tracking her progress for up to two and a half years, they would have placed her squarely in the "Success" column and cheerfully published their conclusion that people like Kate prove it's possible to maintain a significant weight loss over time!

Problem is, if they were like most weight-loss research-ers, they wouldn't have bothered to call back at the end of five years—when they would have learned, both times, that Kate was right around her starting weight again. Just like nearly everyone who diets is after five years. As a group of UCLA researchers led by Traci Mann noted in their 2007 meta-analysis of the scien-tific literature on dieting, "It is important for policymakers to remember that weight regain does not necessarily end when researchers stop following study participants."[1] Fuckin' A.

That review of the weight-loss literature, which looked at dozens of published studies, was utterly damning. In the most rigorously designed studies—long-term, randomized ones—Mann and her colleagues found, "Across these studies, there is not strong evidence for the efficacy of diets in leading to long-term weight loss. In two of the studies, there was not a significant difference between the amount of weight loss main-tained by participants assigned to the diet conditions and those assigned to the control conditions. In the three studies that did find significant differences, the differences were quite small." (The average weight loss in those studies, by the way, was 2.4 pounds.) Among less rigorous studies, the UCLA team noted several "methodological problems"—notably poor follow-up rates, participants self-reporting their weights, researchers confounding the effects of diet with the effects of exercise, and participants going on other diets after the studies ended—that biased "the studies toward showing more effective maintenance of the lost weight." They write:

> In sum, long-term diet studies without control groups find little support for the effectiveness of dieting in leading to sustained weight loss. From one third to two thirds of participants in diets will weigh more four to five years after the diet ends than they did before the diet began. This conclusion comes from studies that are biased toward showing successful weight-loss maintenance by the four factors described above and must be considered a conservative estimate of the percentage of individuals for whom dieting is counterproductive. The true number may well be significantly higher.

Even studies with freakin' everything weighted in favor of a pro-dieting result couldn't get one. One-third to two-thirds of participants ended up fatter.

It gets better. The journal article about the UCLA meta-analysis ultimately reaches this conclusion about all the studies:

In the studies reviewed here, dieters were not able to maintain their weight losses in the long term, and there was not consistent evidence that the diets resulted in significant improvements in their health. In the few cases in which health benefits were shown, it could not be demonstrated that they resulted from dieting, rather than exercise, medication use, or other lifestyle changes. It appears that dieters who manage to sustain a weight loss are the rare exception, rather than the rule. Dieters who gain back more weight than they lost may very well be the norm, rather than an unlucky minority.

In other words, diets don't work.

The one thing Mann and her colleagues did find was that many short-term, randomized trials had significantly greater health outcomes—such as better glycemic control, relief of osteoarthritis symptoms and lower blood pressure—than weight-loss outcomes. It's true: Eating a balanced, nutritious diet and exercising are good for you. But it is stone cold bullshit that those things will make you permanently thin if your body is not so inclined. And eating little enough to lose weight, then gaining it back—as, you'll recall, pretty much everyone does— might just cause its own health problems. What's commonly called "yo-yo dieting" is known as "weight cycling" in medical circles, and here's what the UCLA folks have to say about that: "There is evidence from large-scale observational studies that weight cycling is linked to increased all-cause mortality and to increased mortality from cardiovascular disease. In addition, weight cycling is associated with increased risk for myocardial infarction, stroke, and diabetes, increased high-density lipopro-tein cholesterol, increased systolic and diastolic blood pressure, and even suppressed immune function."

Did you notice how all those icky health issues are the same ones commonly associated with "obesity" and used to scare the capacious pants off us fatties? It's in the papers liter-ally every freakin' day: Fat people suffer from all those diseases and symptoms more than thin people, so you must lose weight! Yeah, except you know what else fat people do more than thin people? Diet. We're just saying.

CORRELATION IS NOT CAUSATION

Even if "obesity-related" illnesses are not actually dieting-related illnesses in disguise—we're no scientists, and among those who are, the jury is very much still out—the fact remains, diets don't work. There is simply no proven, safe way to turn fat people into thin people for more than a few years at a time—and "safe" might just be pushing it where those temporary losses are concerned. So what's a girl who's unhappy with her weight—which, sadly, is the vast majority of us—to do?

Well, first, feel free to get really pissed off while you're let-ting all that sink in. It's not fair that technology hasn't found us a way to make everyone permanently thin, while the culture continues to demand thiness. We have the Internet and organ transplants and cloned sheep, but we still don't have a fucking diet that works? That sucks. But it's the harsh reality, as of 2009. No jet-packs, no hover cars, no diets that work. Right now, all we can do is accept that—and then channel our anger instead toward a culture that keeps browbeating us with the message that thin people are intrinsically better than fat people.

Once you've accepted it, if you're still thinking you'd like to make some "lifestyle changes" anyway, check out the chapters on intuitive eating and exercise, which we discuss in terms of an approach to wellness called Health At Every Size.

CHAPTER TWO

Practice Health At Every Size, Including Yours

There's so much focus on weight loss in this culture that we sometimes forget about the independent benefits of exercise and eating nutritious food—to wit, that they make you feel and function better, mentally and physically. What they usually don't do, however, is make fat people permanently thin, which leads a lot of people to give up on the exercise routines and veggie consumption they started as part of a diet.

Fact is, a sedentary lifestyle and poor eating habits *are* hard on your health—but those things are too often erroneously conflated with fatness. There are people who eat lots of junk food and don't work out, yet never gain a significant amount of weight—don't we all know someone like that? Likewise, there are fat people who do get plenty of exercise and eat their veggies, yet never lose a significant amount of weight. You probably know someone like that, too (you may even be like that), but because we're encouraged so strongly to equate "poor diet and lack of exercise" with "fatness," those people tend to be invisible in this culture. Through our work online, we've met numerous fat vegans, fat athletes, and fat health nuts who all tell the same story: They're accused time and again of lying about what they eat and how much they exercise. According to the prevailing wisdom, if you're fat, you must have an "unhealthy lifestyle," and if you're thin, you probably have a healthy one.

Bullshit. It is entirely possible to be a fat person with a healthy lifestyle—and becoming one of those (if you're not already) is a much more reasonable and achievable goal than becoming a thin person. This is where Health At Every Size (HAES) comes in. HAES is the anti-diet—it's all about treating your body well, regardless of whether you lose weight.

DIETING VERSUS HAES

In a study by scientists at the USDA Agricultural Research Service and the University of California–Davis, seventy-eight obese women were divided into two groups—one following traditional diet and exercise advice, and one following the HAES approach. Here's the difference, according to an article by Marcia Wood in the March 2006 issue of *Agricultural Research*[1]:

> Both groups were instructed in nutrition basics. Women on the conventional diet track were schooled in topics that are typically covered in many popular weight-loss programs, such as how to monitor their weight, control their eating, and exercise briskly.
>
> Meanwhile, their Every Size colleagues learned how to

build their self-esteem; recognize and follow the body's natural, internal cues to hunger and satiety (a feeling of fullness); make healthy choices at mealtimes and in between; and enjoy some form of physical activity—an approach that's different from exercising mainly to lose weight.

Two years later, those practicing HAES had maintained a stable weight over the entire time, whereas the dieters—sing it with us!—lost at first and then regained, ending up right back where they started. As a weight-loss plan, neither HAES nor dieting is effective. But let's look at some of the interesting differences between the two groups.

In answer to all those folks who carp about fat people's cholesterol and blood pressure, first, we should note that all of the women—who were, you'll recall, clinically obese—started out with cholesterol and blood pressure levels in the normal range. But within that range, the HAES women "lowered their total cholesterol and their systolic blood pressure and were able to maintain those reductions for the entire course of the study." The dieters, meanwhile, did not lower their cholesterol at all, and just like their weight, their systolic blood pressure dropped, then rebounded. (That right there is just the kind of correlation between weight loss and a health benefit that's used to drive the "dieting is good for you" myth, by the way. If you take that group independently, it looks pretty simple—you lose weight and your blood pressure goes down; you regain it, and your blood pressure goes back up. But the other group tells a different story: that longer-lasting health benefits can be gained without losing weight at all. Remember that the next time you read that weight loss is connected to some positive health outcome. As we'll discuss later, correlation does not equal causation.)

But wait, there's more! After two years, members of the HAES group were getting almost four times the amount of exercise they'd gotten prior to the study, whereas the dieters hadn't maintained their new exercise routines. The dieters had improved their "eating behaviors" somewhat, but the HAES volunteers had made and sustained more positive changes in that respect. The HAES group also fared better in terms of avoiding eating disordered behavior and managing depression. And most important, writes Wood:

> At the 2-year point, volunteers answered questions about how helpful the program was to them. When asked whether they'd continued to implement some of the tools they'd learned, 89 percent of the Every Size women answered "regularly" or "often." Only 11 percent of the dieters did so.

In other words, if you really want to make long-term "lifestyle changes" to improve your physical and mental health—as opposed to wanting to get thin and *claiming* it's to improve your health— HAES is far more likely to be successful for you than dieting.

WHAT DOES THIS MEAN TO ME?

So what is HAES? Well, it's a lot of things. Two crucial elements of it—finding a form of exercise you enjoy and learning to listen to your own internal hunger cues (intuitive eating)—will be covered in depth in the next two chapters. But basically, HAES is a philosophy, rather than a structured program. It's about listening to your body and focusing on feeling as good as you possibly can. It's about learning to appreciate all the things your body can do and taking care of yourself, rather than trying to change what you look like. It's about being kind to yourself and working within your own limitations—which might include a genetic predisposition to fatness, a disability, or a chronic disease.

The word *health* being part of the name of this philosophy seems to trip a lot of people up, because our cultural image of a "healthy" person is an able-bodied, disease-free gym bunny who lives on tofu and sprouts. You don't have to be that person to practice HAES—it's all about working with, not against, the body and appetites you've got. If you have fibromyalgia, you can't necessarily exercise as much as you'd like to. If you have diabetes or irritable bowel syndrome (IBS), you can't necessarily eat whatever sounds good to you. If you have a demanding job or kids, or are under a lot of stress for other reasons, you might not always be able to carve out the time or emotional energy for yoga class or swimming or buying and cooking a wide variety of foods. But none of that means you automatically flunk HAES—it just means you've got your own individual limitations, as we all do.

And for our money, one of the most important things to remember with regard to HAES—and pretty much everything else in life—is this: Mental health is a big part of health. You definitely don't want to trade beating yourself up about dieting "failures" for beating yourself up about not doing HAES "correctly." The whole point of HAES is to stop beating yourself up about your body—remember how those women in the Every Size group were also given lessons in improving their self-esteem?—and start honoring it. The form that takes will be different for every person, but the basic philosophy is the same: Be kind to yourself.

Now, we're by no means saying you must jump on the HAES train to improve your body image—as we will say over and over in this book, despite what this culture often suggests, health is not a moral imperative. You are not a bad person if you just don't like working out or eating vegetables, if you have priorities other than trying to live to be one hundred, or if you have a disability that keeps you from ever truly feeling "healthy." But we're going to talk a lot about HAES and related concepts here, because both of us found it led to an incredibly important paradigm shift in our lives. When we started looking at exercising and eating our leafy greens as things that actually made us feel better—not just odious crap we did periodically to punish ourselves for being fat—we both started liking our bodies a whole lot more. More even than we did during those phases when we'd temporarily starved ourselves thinner.

CHAPTER THREE

Find a Form of Exercise You Love

Once upon a time, Marianne was checking out a college in Chicago. It's true what they say—it's a very windy city, indeed. (That line about how the nickname refers to loudmouthed politicians and not the weather? Bull pucky.—Kate) It was March, it was forty degrees, and the hotel was far away from everything. One morning she went out wearing several layers of clothing (given how notoriously bad she is at dressing her Floridian body for the actual weather, this is itself kind of amazing) and instead of feeling frozen, she felt invigorated. She wanted to jump up and down. She wanted to spin around in dizzy circles. She wanted to walk really fast to her destination.

And then she was passed by a jogger. And something in her head just clicked: This is why people jog. They do it for the exhilarating rush, for the thrill of moving through space under their own power. The previously elusive concept of a "runner's high" finally made sense.

Wearing stompy black boots and a velvet skirt, Marianne jogged a few steps. It was awesome! It was amazing! Then it was over very quickly because the cold triggered her asthma, and her lungs spasmed something fierce. And that was the last time she thought about jogging for many, many years.

After all, she was fat. Fat people don't jog. Everybody knows that. And, despite positive feedback about her fitness levels from a personal trainer, she didn't really believe she was in good enough shape to jog.

Fast-forward several years. It's 2 a.m., and Marianne's sitting in a very hot and steamy shower, laboring to breathe. She's considering waking her boyfriend up to take her to the hospital. Instead, she finally gets out of the shower and tries to sleep sitting up. The next day, the walk from the parking lot to her desk exhausts her—there just isn't enough oxygen getting into her lungs. Maybe, she was beginning to suspect, her fitness levels really weren't the problem after all.

That's the day she finally broke down and made an appointment with an allergist. That's the day she realized her fat wasn't actually the problem: It was her respiratory system. She wound up on a host of medications to get her allergies and asthma, which had been coconspirators in ravaging her breathing ability, under control.

Weeks later, she was breathing freely, for the first time in pretty much ever. Her boyfriend chased her across a parking lot, playing, and she ran without gasping for air. She stopped in her tracks.

Y'all, she ran across a parking lot—the most meaningful

moments are often insignificant on the surface. And she could still breathe. As cheesy as it sounds, in that moment, she knew she could jog.

Which is precisely what she did on her next trip to the gym.

EXERCISE CAN BE FUN

Now, obviously, jogging isn't for everyone, and some of you probably think she's insane. (Kate does!) The point is, she is fat, and she jogs. This alone would be enough to confuse people who buy into stereotypes of fat people as lazy and sedentary, but her reasons for it might just make their heads explode: She doesn't jog because it will make her thinner (it probably won't—it hasn't yet!) or because it's a "good" thing to do. She does it because of that exhilarating rush she first experienced in Chicago, the thrill of moving through space under her own formidable power. Those things aren't the sole province of skinny gym rats; they can be experienced at any size.

That was a huge revelation to Kate, too, the first time she went to a yoga class. You mean, there's a form of exercise that isn't 5 percent fun and 95 percent excruciating humiliation? There's a form of exercise that can make me feel better when I walk out than I did when I walked in? Where the hell did this come from?

It's our belief that a whole lot of people are sedentary not because they're lazy, but because they truly don't know that exercise is supposed to—and really can—feel good. If you grew up in the "no pain, no gain," culture, abused by gym teachers and ridiculed by your more coordinated peers, it's perfectly logical to strongly associate exercise with pure, unfettered suck. We both did for a long time, before discovering jogging and yoga, respectively (which eventually led to lots of other exercise interests).

And the thing is, those discoveries weren't just a matter of finding out that exercise can be fun; the really life-changing aspect was learning what it was like to inhabit our bodies, instead of just begrudgingly accepting them as the only available form of transportation for our brains. We found out what it felt like when our heart rates increased and what our muscles felt like as they moved us around. We found out how loose a really good stretch could make our legs feel. We found out that movement was a pretty amazing sensation.

EATING LESS, EXERCISING MORE

Like a lot of girls in this culture, we grew up believing our bodies were primarily something for other people to experience externally; exercise was a means of losing weight and therefore looking more acceptable, not something that might be an intrinsically gratifying experience. No one ever taught us there was a point to moving our bodies if it didn't cause weight loss. Sure, we knew some people really seemed to enjoy sports as recreation, but hoo boy, we weren't among them. And sure, plenty of people gave lip service to the idea of exercising "for your health," but what that really meant was "to lose weight." Fat was bad and unhealthy. Exercise made it go away. That. Was. All.

So if we exercised and didn't lose weight, there was no god-damned reason to keep it up, obviously. We weren't getting any "healthier" or any prettier, and it literally did not occur to us to consider how our bodies actually felt when we exercised. If we noticed anything at all, it was buried under the expectation that we would feel that way all the time when we were thin. Our bodies would finally feel good when they were thin—never mind that our bodies were feeling pretty great when we were fat. When we exercised, there was only one thought in our minds: "If I keep this up for a really long time, I will be thin."

And of course that thought was immediately followed by, "And if I work even harder, I'll be thin a little sooner!"—which meant we often overexerted ourselves, further cementing the mental association of exercise with pain. Pushing your limits within reason can be enjoyable, but for a long time, we had no idea what was reasonable; we just thought thin people must be in pain pretty much all the time, and we apparently weren't tough enough to cope with that. We didn't realize that overextending yourself when you are exercising can cause health problems that never existed for you before! Obviously all those feelings of discomfort were because we were fat, we thought, and then we pushed ourselves even harder, making ourselves feel even worse.

When you think of exercise strictly as some sort of atone-ment for the sin of your fatness, something you must do to become socially acceptable, of course you're going to get sick of it (or injure yourself) and give up sooner rather than later. Sure, some people of a more Puritanical bent might find shame to be a powerful motivator, but most of us don't. A 2007 study published in the *American Journal of Preventive Medicine* found that among teenagers, a history of being teased about their bodies was one of the strongest predictors of both eating disordered behavior and excess weight. Not only did body shame encourage kids to starve themselves or binge, it made them fatter anyway.[1]

More recently, researchers who looked at a group of about 170,000 American adults found that the difference between actual weight and perceived ideal weight was a better barometer of physical and mental health than one's BMI score—in other words, feeling too fat is worse for your health than being fat.[2] So contrary to popular opinion, which holds that if fat people aren't marginalized, they'll see no reason to lose weight and thus will cost the health care system buckets of money and cause the downfall of Western civilization, and on and on and on, shame and self-loathing do not make people want to take better care of their bodies. And why would they? Who do you treat better—your best friend or your worst enemy? This should be a flippin' no-brainer.

Yet doing exercise you enjoy, because you enjoy it, without giving a rat's ass about whether you lose weight, is still a pretty radical idea for most people. Which is absurd, considering the studies that have shown improving your fitness level has enormous health benefits even if you remain fat. Our culture and media are so obsessed with weight loss that this fact too easily gets lost in the shuffle. But researchers have found that fit adults live longer than unfit ones, irrespective of body weight.[3]

Because we know diets don't work for the vast majority of

people, fat and fit is the best a lot of us can hope for. And everyone agrees that's at least healthier than fat and unfit (though you may want to reread the chapter on HAES before you start using relative health to judge people). So what's the problem with telling people that exercise is a good thing, whether they lose weight or not? (We'll actually attempt to answer that question later, but for now, just consider it rhetorical and nod along with us.)

DID YOU SAY FUN?

Now that that's out of our systems, let's get back to the "exercise is fun" part. We will grant you that not every form of movement is fun for every person. Kate hates jogging as much as Marianne loves it. (Brisk walking provides all the fun with none of the boob and knee pain, people.) And for as much as Kate loves yoga, she also knows at least half a dozen people who find it boring beyond belief. Ditto Pilates, which she just recently got into (and which Marianne hates). We both enjoy swimming and water aerobics but have loads of friends who believe nothing involving a bathing suit could possibly be a positive experience. You don't have to love what we love, or what your best friend or partner loves, or whatever *Glamour* tells you is the hottest new fitness trend. You just have to find out what form(s) of exercise you love.

And when you find that thing or things, you won't need any tips on sticking with a routine or tricking yourself into dragging your butt to the gym. When you love doing something, you want to do it. Go figure! And, if you miss some time at yoga class because life got in the way, you start to miss the activity—which motivates you to start doing it again. Crazy, huh? Why, it's almost like people, left to their own devices, will seek pleasure and avoid pain! (That's the last time you'll hear us quote Freud, promise, but he had a point there.)

The bad news is, figuring out which physical activities give you that giddy, exhilarated feeling instead of leaving you humiliated and in pain can only be done by trial and error. A good start is reading up on the activity that interests you and seriously considering whether or not you can see yourself loving it. There will still be errors. And those errors, of course, will be yet more crappy exercise experiences, which might leave you feeling like you were right all along: Working out is not for you, period. In that case, we'd just encourage you to try one more class. One more sport. One more walk. And then one more, if that one sucks, too. It's kind of like dating, really; the bad ones can be so bad that you want to give up altogether, but when you find the one you're crazy about, you'll know it was all worth it.

CHAPTER FOUR

Practice Intuitive Eating

It's 2:30 in the afternoon, and your body, it seems, has declared war on you. You can't focus, your head hurts, and your stomach is cramping up. Why is this happening? You had breakfast. Oh, wait, instead you stopped and got coffee on your way to work. Well, you had lunch. . . . But, hey, that microwave meal only had 260 calories in it. It would be easy to go to the vending machine, but you're being good. You'll just fill up your trusty water bottle or grab a diet soda and muscle through the hunger. Food is for the weak!

Yeah, because that is *so* healthy.

But that's how millions of American women approach eating every day. Even though diets don't work. Even though dieting and disordered eating are virtually the same thing—when a thin person obsessively restricts calories and compulsively exercises, we call it anorexia, but when a fat person does those things, we call it "taking good care of her body!" Our national obsession with shrinking—which is a vile term but at least honest—has people treating hunger as though it is optional.

Let's put this simply: If you don't eat, you die. Because of this, the body has developed a handy little signal to let you know your body needs fuel. That signal is hunger. That fuel is food. When you tell hunger to shut up, that's when all those fun symptoms of low blood sugar appear. Don't believe me? Skip breakfast, eat one of those tiny diet meals for lunch, and then ask your coworkers (the honest ones who aren't afraid of you) whether they think you ought to eat something there, Grumpasaurus.

And so we are proud to present to you, for the low, low cost of free (well, if you're reading a library copy or thumbing through this chapter in a bookstore), the Harding-Kirby Lifetime Diet Plan: Eat what you're hungry for when you're hungry for it, and stop when you're full. Period.

We can hear your objections from here, and we'll get to that in a minute. But first, we need to tell you a little more about this plan.

I'M STILL HUNGRY

The Harding-Kirby Lifetime Diet Plan, we must confess, isn't an idea we came up with all on our own. It's actually called intuitive eating or "demand feeding" (which is also, we understand, a very popular method of feeding babies), and it means learning to interpret the signals your body is sending you, and then honoring those signals by eating something.

It also means there is no such thing as good food and bad food. If you want an apple, you should eat the apple. If you want a cookie, you should eat the cookie. You absolutely should not eat the apple if you want a cookie, just because you are trying to be virtuous. There is no virtue in self-deprivation, unless you belong to a religious order that demands that sort of thing—and even they would probably be horrified by the self-abnegation that dieters put themselves through.

Eating when you are hungry, until you are full, has become a radical act. You can't go anywhere, including a lot of restaurants, without being slapped in the face by "healthy" options that are anything but. From hundred-calorie snack packs at the grocery store to menus with a special Atkins section, you are being fed the message that your hunger can't be trusted. Someone else—a doctor, a weight-loss counselor, a manufacturer of processed foods—must be in charge of telling you what and how much to eat, 'cause left to your own devices, you'll just screw it all up.

Funny, it's the diet industry that we don't trust. Our hunger hasn't steered us wrong yet.

Still confused? Well, as bloggers, we figure the best thing to do here is offer a list of frequently asked questions.

1. Wait, what? Intuitive eating?

Intuitive eating is, in its simplest form, eating what you want to eat when you are hungry. The most revolutionary thing it means, from the standpoint of our diet culture, is that there is no such thing as *good* food and *bad* food. There is just food. Although IntuitiveEating.com is kind of New Agey froufrou with pictures of flowers and whatnot, it's a good intro to the concept. In fact, we will quote our favorite part of their site:

> Reject the Diet Mentality: Throw out the diet books and magazine articles that offer you false hope of losing weight quickly, easily, and permanently. Get angry at the lies that have led you to feel as if you were a failure every time a new diet stopped working and you gained back all of the weight. If you allow even one small hope to linger that a new and better diet might be lurking around the corner, it will prevent you from being free to rediscover Intuitive Eating.

> Get angry, people!

2. What if I only want to eat bad things?

Again, There are no such things as good food and bad food. One of the tricky things about transitioning to intuitive eating is that you might just go a little nuts from the freedom initially. Once the Twizzlers are not off-limits, you may very well want to eat nothing but Twizzlers. That might even be the only message you hear from your body at first, which can certainly make you question the wisdom of listening to it.

But this isn't because Twizzlers (cheesecake/pizza/fries/whatev) are actually that awesome, or because your body doesn't really know what it wants. It's because there is nothing more delicious than the forbidden. And really, truly convincing your-self that no foods are—or should be—forbidden is quite pos-sibly the most difficult part of the Harding-Kirby Lifetime Diet Plan. We're so conditioned to believe not only that broccoli is good for us and ice cream is not, but that broccoli will make us better people, and ice cream will make us worse. You're going to have to remind yourself over and over that this is bullshit.

For starters, ice cream is full of protein, calcium, and vita-min A. If your blood sugar is low, your body will welcome the carbs in it. Likewise, if you're really hungry, your body will welcome the filling fat. Does this mean ice cream is "good"? No. It means ice cream is food, which is morally neutral. Eat-ing ice cream is not actually equivalent, health-wise, to pouring battery acid down your throat, no matter how much people who dispense dieting advice might like you to believe that it is. It is fueling your body—and if what your body really needs at a given moment is a big dose of calcium or protein, then ice cream is actually a much better choice at that moment than broccoli would be.

3. But what if I only crave "bad" foods?

Many people, when they begin to practice intuitive eating, gravitate toward the foods they've been taught to see as "bad," because suddenly having permission to eat them (as if adults should need permission to eat food!) feels so exciting.

It passes. Because the whole point here is learning to listen to your body, you just need to trust that your body will eventually say, "Hey, I'm sick of ice cream now, and I'd really like something green or fruity." It will. We swear.

So this brings us to the number one piece of advice we have regarding most questions about intuitive eating: Just ride it out and eat what you want when you are hungry for it. Eventually, you'll learn to understand your body's messages and that you feel better if you listen to them. There is no set time limit for this process.

4. What if I never know what I want to eat?

This is, once you commit to it, one of the hardest parts of intuitive eating. Sometimes you are super clear that you want beef teriyaki, and you want it now. But other times you know you're hungry and you should eat and . . .

At that point you have to stop playing What Do I Want To Eat. It is okay not to figure it out every time. The important thing in these moments is to know that you are hungry and to eat something. You aren't a toddler who has to be coaxed to eat by your favorite foods. Eat something simple, something you know will satisfy you. Maybe you'll realize halfway through that what you really wanted was something else entirely. You'll learn from that and take it into account next time you are hungry.

5. What if I don't get hungry?

Marianne was—and sometimes still is—the worst about this. At the height of her disordered eating, she'd skip meals for days because she just didn't feel hungry. The thought of food made her ill. Of course it did! She'd been starving herself, and introducing typical college food to her system was a recipe for intestinal distress.

Kate, meanwhile, didn't even realize how often she got truly hungry until she started practicing intuitive eating. Since high school, she'd been having coffee for breakfast and had come to think of herself as someone who "just doesn't get hungry in the morning." Yeah, that was crap. She got hungry in the morning—she just ignored it. Which meant she was ravenous by lunch, and the only message she could hear from her body was, "Fill me up, now!" Turns out, when she has oatmeal and berries or a bagel or a real Egg McMuffin for breakfast, then at lunch she might crave any number of different foods, instead of just the largest amount of fat in the quickest delivery system possible. Go figure!

When you begin to eat on a regular basis, your body begins to expect food. Both of us now know when we've gone too long without eating, because our bodies will throw a damn fit. We could push past that, sure, but why would we want to? Why would you?

6. How can I crave foods I've never tried before? / What about variety?

The short and easy answer is this: You try new things. We try them when they are there, or when we're trying a new recipe, or whenever we're feeling adventurous. Intuitive eating doesn't mean feeling absolutely rapturous about every single thing you eat, or positive it's precisely what your body was craving—it just means eating what sounds good, whenever you're hungry. And to us, lots of things we've never eaten before can sound good, especially if they're paired with more familiar yums.

Some people are far more adventurous than others, and either end of the spectrum (and, of course, everything in the middle) is okay. You probably aren't going to crave something you've never tried, but since not every meal is going to answer a specific "I want this plus this plus this" formula, you have a lot of room to work.

7. Will intuitive eating help me lose weight?

Maybe, maybe not. Intuitive eating isn't meant to affect your weight in a deliberate way. You can say you are eating intuitively with the intention of losing weight but, frankly, we're not sure how that would work, given the radical philosophical disconnect there. Weight-loss dieting is about rules and restrictions; intuitive eating is about letting go of those things.

It's possible, if you've been consistently overeating up until now, that you've gotten beyond your natural weight range, and once you've been eating intuitively for a while, your body will find that range again. But basically, that range is what it is—and it's fucking stubborn. You have to eat a lot to get beyond it, and pretty much starve yourself to get under it. Unless you're currently bingeing or dieting, you're probably already somewhere in that twenty to thirty pound range your body thinks is right for you—which means substantial weight loss is highly unlikely.

It's kinda like this: Have you ever met one of those annoying Westerners who's essentially taken up Buddhism as a hobby and self-identifies as a Very Serious Religious Person with a Deep Understanding of Eastern Philosophy? And you know how Buddhism is fundamentally about releasing your attachments to earthly things, but said annoying Westerners inevitably recommend Buddhism because it's made their lives—their distinctly earthly lives—so much better? Well, approaching intuitive eating with an eye to weight loss is sort of like becoming a Buddhist in hopes that your newfound calmness and insight will help earn you a promotion so you can buy an awesome house. It's not supposed to be about getting something you haven't got; it's about accepting and honoring what is.

8. How am I supposed to afford this?

Our grocery bills have gone down since we started intuitive eating. We don't waste so much money on food we're not going to eat. We spend less on eating out. We don't overbuy in the hopes that OMG *something* will appeal to us at some point. We just go to the grocery store a lot more often. (Okay, Marianne does. Kate still gets a lot of takeout.)

However, if you're poor or very poor, eating intuitively can be nigh unto inaccessible; what your body craves won't always be what you can afford. We don't think this is a failure of the concept of intuitive eating, but a failure of our society, on a lot of levels. If you don't have a grocery store in your neighborhood—as many people living in lower-income communities don't—whether or not you can afford a fresh avocado is kind of beside the point. You don't have access. Disordered eating knows no socioeconomic boundaries, but one of the best ways around it does.

There are probably ways to incorporate intuitive eating into a very restricted budget, but we know it can be difficult. We've heard from several readers who say they'd love to eat intuitively, but sometimes simply cannot fit much beyond rice, pasta, and peanut butter into the budget. So all we can really offer is our best advice about eating, exercising, shopping, loving, and life in general: Do what you can do with what you've got, and don't beat yourself up about doing it "wrong."

9. How am I supposed to do this with a partner/family/kids?

Do you eat every single morsel of food that you have in a day with someone else? If your answer is yes, it might be a little difficult, but through the magic of compromise and thinking about food in new ways, this can be worked out. If you answered no, it might still be a little difficult, but through the magic of compromise and thinking about food in new ways, this can be worked out.

See, as we've said before, not every meal is going to be a revelation. Sometimes, you are just going to feel like "crunchy" or "meaty sauce" or "hot" or "eaten with my fingers" or any number of other vague things. Somewhere in there you will find something that will satisfy both you and your partner, maybe even your kids.

But let's be real here: Kids are a pain in the ass to feed, unless you're one of those "You can eat what I made or go to bed hungry!" parents. We've observed that that child-rearing style is not so much in vogue these days, so we're going to operate on the assumption that you're already thinking, if not agonizing, about what you'll give the kids to eat at any given meal without starving them, stuffing them, or giving them scurvy.

We're just telling you to ask yourself the same question.

Sometimes, like we've said, the answer is that you compromise. It's more complicated with kids than if you're just talking about two adults who can either compromise or fix their own dinner. Obviously no one wants to prepare four different meals. But, at the same time, if you're buying what we're selling here, you're going to want to teach your kids to eat intuitively—which means teaching them to be aware of and honor their hunger. That means not telling your kids they're *really* thirsty or bored or whatever when they say they are hungry. If your child wants nothing but raisins for a week and you have a week's supply of raisins, go ahead and let them see what happens when you eat nothing but raisins for a week (Marianne can speak from her own childhood experience: nothing good). Teaching your kids to eat intuitively means trusting them when they tell you about their food experiences. Respect their hunger. Respect that their hunger is different from your own.

But at the same time, if everyone in the family will agree to eat a tuna casserole, even though it's not what any one of you is dying for, that casserole will do just fine. Not every meal has to be perfect or memorable. It just has to be satisfying.

10. What if I am committed to eating ethically/locally/non-meatily?

That's awesome! You're a much better person than we are! And you, too, can eat intuitively.

Intuitive eating doesn't mean you are blindly at the mercy of your cravings. You are an adult, and you get to make the decisions here. So if your body is craving a rare steak, but you are a committed vegan, it's okay! You don't have to go out and eat the rare steak. But you might want to load up on veggies that are high in iron. Sometimes we crave things our brain identifies as a specific food when really we're craving some specific nutrient.

And sometimes, once again, you just have to compromise. Kate, in Chicago, is a big fan of farmers' markets in the summer, but in the winter, the produce she eats sure ain't local. She's happy enough to settle for imported fruit and frozen veggies during the cold months; if you're more of a purist, you might want to take a tip from Marianne's great-grandmother and make preserves or dehydrate fruit when it's in season. If you're even more hard-core than that, Marianne also recommends moving to Florida, where she has access to local fresh fruits and veggies year-round. (Bitch.) The degree to which you're willing to compromise is up to you. Just remember the cardinal rule: Do what you can do with what you've got, and don't beat yourself up.

11. What if I just don't stop eating?

This is a tough one to answer. It could be a lot of different things, and some of those might be things we're not qualified to diagnose. We're going to answer this question assuming that you don't actually suffer from Binge Eating Disorder (BED), which is a whole different ball of wax from occasionally eating until you need to undo your belt buckle. If you think you might suffer from BED, you can find more information at the National Health Information Center (mentalhealth.samhsa.gov) or the National Eating Disorders Association (nationaleatingdisorders.org).

If you don't, though, you're probably just afraid you won't stop eating—and you're probably wrong.

Figuring out what you're hungry for and how hungry you are after a lifetime of being told you are always too hungry for the wrong foods, is a bitch. As we've said, we both still struggle with it—with the fear of deprivation, with baggage about "good" and "bad" foods, with feeling like every meal must contain all of the food groups. So trying to listen to our bodies instead of the voices in our heads involves a lot of conscious effort—which is exactly what you're trying to drop by, you know, listening to your body. It will get easier.

Maybe the best way to stop feeling as if you're going to devour the world is to actually go ahead and try to devour the world. Because the first thing you'll realize is that you can't. And the next thing you'll realize is that you don't really want to. And once you get to that point, you might actually have a prayer of understanding your own internal hunger cues.

12. Why is this so hard?

Because it means we have to take a lot of personal responsibility for our own food choices, instead of farming them out to the "experts." Because we are so disconnected from our own hunger and hunger signals. Because it takes time and energy and effort to procure and prepare foods; even though we *have* to eat, we can still be resentful of the process and not feel deserving of that much time, energy, and effort. Because it takes creativity and compromise to eat intuitively, especially if you have a family. Because of the way our cultures have raised us to relate (or not) with food. Because it means we actually might enjoy our food when we are already stereotyped as fat and gluttonous. Because of all sorts of things.

But it is better than the alternative, which is acting as though feeding ourselves decently requires a PhD in nutrition. Our bodies have more wisdom than we give them credit for. It's time to learn how to give your body some credit.

PART TWO

{ **Mental Health** }

CHAPTER FIVE

If You Think You Might Be Suffering from Depression, Get Help

Sometimes you just feel sad. Sad and fat and horrible and like you just aren't worth taking care of. We've all had those days when getting out of bed has been a Herculean task and actually accomplishing anything is twice as hard. On days like that, Marianne likes to buy herself some new lip gloss or just take a hot bath with a romance novel. Kate likes to hang out with friends, do yoga, or just lie in bed feeling sorry for herself. (Hey, sometimes it works.)

But some days just aren't so simple. When days like that turn into weeks and then into months, depression might be a factor.

According to the National Institute of Mental Health, approximately 20.9 million Americans suffer from a mood disorder such as major or minor depression, or bipolar disorder. These disorders can make it even more difficult for anyone to think positively and take care of herself, but if you already struggle with body image issues, the negative thinking that depression naturally fosters can make you flat-out hate yourself.

Furthermore, lethargy, apathy, and disruption of sleep patterns—all symptoms of depression—make it difficult to function, to say the least. When everything in your life feels like it is going wrong (and that it is your fault for sucking so much), treating yourself well takes a backseat to just surviving. And it's kind of impossible to fight off the societal message that your body is all wrong when your own brain is sending you that message, too. That's why it's important to get help if you think you might have a mood disorder such as depression. You have enough on your mental plate without adding in the extra fun of a chemical imbalance.

Kate saw her first psychologist when she was sixteen, and he and later talk-doctors all agreed that she suffered from depression. Unfortunately, being psychologists and not psychiatrists, they couldn't prescribe medication—and they weren't sure she needed it anyway. Kate's a really reactive person. When things are going well, she's pretty chipper, but when she's stressed out, she can sink into an unshakeable black funk very fast. For a long time, both she and her therapists assumed that this meant she only suffered from situational depression, not that she had a permanent imbalance going on in her head. But then, when she was thirty-one, she was so tired of slipping into those funks, she decided she wanted to try antidepressants to see if they'd make any difference.

And, well, put it this way: After years of drifting and dreaming about a writing career, within two years of starting on antidepression meds, she founded a blog that would garner thousands of daily readers and major media attention, got on the payroll at her favorite online magazine (Salon.com), secured literary representation, and, oh yeah, sold this book you're reading (with a little help from Marianne). Antidepressants aren't right for everyone—and even if they are, finding the right drug can take some trial and error—but treating depression can remove a whole lot of obstacles in the way of your feeling like your best self.

Marianne, instead of dealing with depression per se, has been diagnosed as bipolar type II. One defining characteristic of this disorder can be rapid cycling—which means that sometimes Marianne would feel great and sometimes . . . not so much. During hypomanic periods, she was productive, energetic, creative, and very active. During depressive phases . . . again, not so much.

Can you guess how her body image cycled right along with her moods?

Getting treatment helped Marianne think rationally about body image, and it also allowed her to start seriously working on getting over her body hate. It's still a struggle when the depression comes to town, but she's managed to build a foundation—and she knows that the depression is a temporary thing.

HOW DO YOU KNOW IF YOU'RE DEPRESSED?

So how do you know you have depression? According to the fourth edition of the *Diagnostic and Statistical Manual of Mental Disorders*, if you experience the following symptoms—especially either of the first two—you are probably dealing with depression. If you look at this list and see yourself reflected there, it is a good idea to contact your doctor. (And if you're feeling suicidal, please tell someone—anyone.)

- Feelings of sadness or the seeming inability to feel emotion (emptiness).

- A decrease in the amount of interest or pleasure in all, or almost all, daily activities.

- Changing appetite and marked weight gain or loss.

- Disturbed sleep patterns, such as insomnia, loss of REM sleep, or excessive sleep (hypersomnia).

- Fatigue, mental or physical; also loss of energy.

- Intense feelings of guilt, nervousness, helplessness, hopelessness, worthlessness, isolation/loneliness and/or anxiety.

- Trouble concentrating, keeping focused, or making decisions or a generalized slowing and worsening of cognition, including memory.

- Recurrent thoughts of death (not just fear of dying), desire to just "lie down and die" or "stop breathing," recurrent suicidal thoughts without a specific plan, or a suicide attempt or a specific plan for completing suicide.

One final point about depression and body image. Feeling shitty in general, not just about your body, can make you want to diet, even if you know that's not a long-term solution to pretty much anything. Dieting is hard, but compared to a lot of other things—coping with work or family stress, trying to fix a broken relationship, or going through whatever steps are necessary to get help for suspected depression—it's actually pretty easy. Or at least, it's straightforward. You get a plan, you stick to it, you see results. At first. And if you're disgusted with yourself for being fat, losing weight actually can help you feel better and improve your body image. At first. It also makes you feel like you've taken control of at least one part of your life. At first.

So, when everything's going wrong, dieting can seem like an appealing panacea. As S. C. Wooley and D. M. Garner—two prominent researchers who have studied and written about the ineffectiveness of dieting—wrote in the *Journal of the American Dietetic Association* in 1991:

> Obese patients are often encouraged to believe that weight loss is an appropriate way to combat depression, save a failing marriage, or increase the chance of career success. The irrationality of hopes pinned on weight loss is so striking that dieting might almost be likened to superstitious behavior. . . . Passing from childhood into adolescence, leaving home, marrying, starting a new job, having a baby, experiencing marital difficulties, adjusting to children leaving home, and growing old—all these life situations may become unexamined reasons to diet. In other instances, concerns over weight mask even more serious problems.[1]

A lot of fat (and even not-so-fat) women and men believe on some level that their problems will be solved if they just lose some weight—it will automatically make them healthier, prouder, and happier. But if you suffer from clinical depression, becoming thin will not lift you out of it. That's why we've devoted a whole chapter to this topic. About 9.5 percent of the population—the number of Americans thought to have mood disorders—may not seem like a lot of people, but we know so many people personally and among our readers whose depression went untreated for years because they always believed they'd be happy if they just weren't so fat. Thinness will not bring you happiness, but getting checked out for problems that go beyond "the blues" just might.

CHAPTER SIX

Find Body-Positive Doctors
and Go to Them

Marianne's favorite time of year isn't a season or a holiday. Nope, she loves going to her annual eye exam. And not just because she loves getting new glasses.

No, Marianne loves going to the eye doctor, because for years and years and years, the eye doctor was the one doctor she could go to who wouldn't mention her weight. Has anyone blamed astigmatism on being fat? (Wait, we probably shouldn't give them any ideas.)

Unfortunately, going to just the eye doctor doesn't cut it. We all need to go to other doctors, the kind who take your blood pressure and listen to your heart and, yes, often say things like, "What are we going to do about your weight?" as if they'll actually be participating in the process of "doing something about it."

Until recently, Marianne resisted finding one of those. The last time she had gone to the doctor, the man told her a small head of broccoli, purchased to go along with every dinner, instead ought to last her an entire week *as* dinner. Even though she wasn't eating much else. Because, you know, starvation diets are so healthy. (Also, wouldn't the broccoli be kind of nasty after a week?) Marianne never went back to that doctor but she didn't go to any other doctors (except the eye doctor), either.

For the record, this is not a good way to approach your health.

Fast-forward several years, and Marianne is sicker than she has ever been. Remember that story from the exercise chapter about her sitting in the shower in the middle of the night, wondering if she needed to go to the emergency room? Her asthma and allergies had gotten that bad because the only thing more terrifying than not being able to breathe was the thought of finding a new doctor. She was terrified of being yelled at, of her fat being blamed for her allergies (which had happened before), and of the doctor not taking her seriously.

I'M AFRAID

If you find yourself just as frightened as Marianne was by the prospect of going to a new physician, you're not crazy. It is incredibly common for fat people to be mistreated at the hands of their doctors. Writing in the *Permanente Journal* in 2003, obesity researchers Kelly Brownell and Rebecca Puhl examined several studies that attempted to measure weight-based discrimination by health care professionals, revealing "explicit negative attitudes about obesity among physicians, nurses, dieticians, and medical students. These attitudes include: obese people lack self-control and are lazy, obesity is caused by character flaws, and failure to lose weight is due only to noncompliance."[1] In one study, 24 percent of nurses surveyed reported feeling "repulsed" by obese patients. And a study using the Implicit Associations Test—a tool for determining unconscious prejudices—found that even doctors who did not outwardly seem to hold negative feelings toward fat folks likely still believed the stereotypes deep down—which is to say, as Brownell and Puhl put it, "societal anti-fat attitudes are so pervasive that even those who dedicate their lives to treating obesity aren't immune from these attitudes, despite wishing to avoid prejudice."

When there's a one in four chance that the nurse who weighs you will find you repulsive and the physician who treats you is likely to think you're lazy and out of control (even if she doesn't think she's biased), going to the doctor becomes more than just your garden variety pain in the ass. It can be emotionally treacherous.

It can be physically treacherous, too. In 2007, Kate cofounded a website called First, Do No Harm: Real Stories of Fat Prejudice in Health Care (fathealth.org), where readers send in their own experiences of being neglected, mistreated, and disbelieved by doctors who couldn't see past their weight. Some of these anecdotes make Marianne's experience look pretty tame, including:

- A woman who gained seventy pounds—a third of her body weight—in a year, and was told by physicians that she must be eating too much and exercising too little, period. It turned out she had a thyroid tumor.

- A woman who swims and lifts weights regularly, who saw a doctor regarding a bout of severe back pain. He blamed the pain on her weight and only prescribed dieting and more exercise. She tried to comply, drastically reducing her calorie intake (she was in too much pain to work out by that point) but also saw a physiotherapist, who actually listened to her and identified the real problem: She'd torn a muscle while lifting weights, and her back had locked up to, as she put it, force her to lie still and heal.

- A woman who was handed a Weight Watchers pamphlet by a nurse while she was in the ER with appendicitis.

- A woman with polycystic ovarian syndrome (PCOS)—one symptom of which is weight gain—whose fertility doctor told her "it would be unethical" to help her get pregnant, unless she lost weight.

These stories are all too common. Fat people don't even get to have normal illnesses or accidents just like thin people, you see. Even if we hurt ourselves working out, or take a spill on some ice, well, that's because we're fat and clumsy. Rx: Lose weight. It can start to seem like losing weight is always the only remedy a doctor will offer—or at least inevitably the first prescription, regardless of the patient's complaint.

As if that weren't bad enough, fat people have also been denied transplants, joint replacements, and elective surgery, because, the thinking goes, such interventions will be wasted on us and/or too difficult for the doctors to perform.[2] In 2007, a

British woman named Anjelica Allan was denied a hip replacement for being six pounds "overweight"—and smaller than the
national average for women, no less. (Fortunately, the national
media fuss shamed the Lincolnshire Primary Care Trust into
admitting they denied operations to people with BMI scores over
thirty simply to cut costs, and Allan eventually got her new hip.[3])
No one ever answers how people with excruciating joint pain—
especially those with a lot more than six pounds to lose—are
supposed to drop the weight, when their disabilities presumably
prevent them from exercising. Starvation, apparently?

What about people who need organ transplants—do we
really think they're going to be hitting the gym with a renewed
fervor after being told they can't have lifesaving surgery? Is there
a "lite" version of IV feeding? Instead of the medical community learning new techniques for operating on fat bodies, say,
or studying why obese patients are more likely to have adverse
outcomes after surgery (these are the reasons usually given for
handing a kidney to a thin person farther down the list), the
onus is on us to lose weight if we want to deserve proper treatment. Complete health care, evidently, is something you have
to earn—and too many physicians believe that fat folks just
aren't working hard enough.

It's no wonder, then, that one study mentioned by Brownell
and Puhl found "more than 12 percent of women indicated
they delayed or canceled physician appointments because of
weight concerns. In addition, 32 percent of women with BMI
over twenty-seven and 55 percent of women with BMI over
thirty-five delayed or canceled visits because they knew they

would be weighed. The most common reason for delaying appointments was *embarrassment about weight*."[4] (Emphasis ours.) You're not silly, crazy, or alone if you're afraid a doctor visit will involve a humiliating lecture on your weight at best and inadequate care at worst. It's a real problem.

FINDING A FAT-FRIENDLY PHYSICIAN

Of course the last thing you need when you're trying to make peace with your own body is someone in a white coat telling you that you need to diet. That's some depressing shit, but here comes the good news. Believe it or not, many doctors are realistic about the success rates of weight-loss programs, and an increasing number of them practice and encourage a Health At Every Size approach to wellness. (See Chapter 2.)

Marianne finally got lucky after that horrible middle-of-the-night shower incident. She found an allergist who actually treated her allergies, and that gave her the confidence to find a GP and an ob-gyn. None of them have ever recommended she lose weight. None of them have ever blamed a medical complaint on her fat. None of them have ever treated Marianne with anything other than kindness and respect.

But what about you? If you are avoiding the doctor because you think they will yell at you or because, worst of all, you believe you don't deserve good treatment, you do have options.

- **First, be prepared to look for a doctor before you need one.** When you've been struck with the death flu and you are desperate for care, your standards might not be quite as exacting. Start talking to doctors when you are feeling good, both physically and mentally.

- **Do some research.** Ask friends, especially fat friends, what doctors they go to and pay attention to the answers. If your friends suggest their doctors but also say, "Oh, they only yell at me every so often," you probably ought to skip making an appointment. Check out some of the resources listed in the back of this book to find HAES-friendly doctors. These resources—notably the Fat-Friendly Health Professionals List maintained by Stef at Cat-and-Dragon.com—are living documents, being updated all the time. If there's not a doctor listed in your area, keep checking back.

- **When you call a doctor's office, talk to the nurse or receptionist who answers the phone. Ask them if they support the practice of HAES.** Inquire about the doctor's policies on dieting. If the office doesn't sound like a friendly and supportive environment, it's time to call the next doctor on your list.

- **When you've found a doctor that seems awesome, schedule an appointment for a consult.** Go in and talk to the doctor. Ask whatever questions are concerning you; tell the doctor you don't want to be weighed (if you don't want to be weighed) and see how she or he responds. You might want to take a letter you've written, expressing your expectations and some of your background with doctors.

- **And, once you have chosen a doctor, continue to insist on high standards of treatment.** Your doctor is working for you. If you think the doctor is dismissing a concern, call him or her on it. We're all human, so we aren't saying that you need to storm out in a fit of outrage if the doctor suggests upping your vitamin C intake. But it is your doctor's job to take you and your health seriously.

Once you've found a good doctor, it's your job to take her or him seriously as well. If you've injured your knee and the doc wants you to wear a brace because your weight might place undue strain on it, that's a pretty fair concern. If he needs to know your weight to determine the correct dosage of a medication, it's time to step up on the scale. (You can always stand backward and ask them not to tell you what you weigh, if you think the number will make you crazy.) If your doctor suddenly says you might want to consider eating more vegetables, ask her why, instead of reacting with knee-jerk defensiveness.

Now, sometimes, you wind up with a doctor that seems decent but then you go in for a routine visit and leave in tears. What do you do then? First of all, don't go back. And you tell them why. (A good rule of thumb is that unless you've gotten a devastating diagnosis—and we hope you never do!—you should not find yourself crying about what happened at the doctor's office.) Second, file a complaint with the state medical board. The procedure is state-specific, but you can easily find the relevant websites online. For readers outside of the United States, chances are good that your local doctors are governed by some sort of similar board. Seek out that board and their manner of handling complaints.

Remember that doctor who suggested Marianne needed to go on a starvation diet? She filed a complaint against him. She knew there was only a small chance that he would be disciplined for his crazy talk, but it was worth the effort to alert future potential patients to the doctor's practices. Although complaints are not searchable, if a doctor receives enough, then that doctor will be investigated and disciplined. And you can check with your local medical board to find out if a doctor has had disciplinary action brought against him (and for what reason) in the past.

The most effective weapon we have against doctors who treat us like crap is our voices. If we are vocal, to medical boards and to each other, about discriminatory and neglectful treatment, then maybe someday our children or grandchildren won't have to worry about being offered weight-loss surgery brochures when they get strep throat.

Fat Hatred Kills

by Barbara Benesch-Granberg

Note: Barbara's mother died on May 1, 2007, and this essay was written about two months later.

My mother and I had a very difficult relationship for a long time, and though we weren't fighting when she died, we weren't exactly on speaking terms, either. That's difficult for me to cope with.

But people understand that. People get that. And so a lot of people have been very kind and reassuring, reminding me that even if we never could seem to just talk to each other, she knew I loved her just as I knew she loved me.

What's more difficult for me to cope with is the anger.

It's hard to even know where to begin, to express this white-hot rage I carry. And what's extra-hard about it is that I can't really talk to many people about it. I've tried, but most of the responses I've gotten only serve to piss me off more.

See, this is what I'm pissed off about: My mom is dead not because she was fat, but because of how she was *treated* for being fat.

She died at home, alone, from a blood clot that had formed in one of her legs and traveled to her lungs, killing her. The coroner's report says that she had deep vein thrombosis (DVT) and probably had been dealing with it for some time. In fact, the coroner said that over the past year or so, when she kept having "asthma attacks" that weren't helped by her inhaler, they were actually very small blood clots blocking parts of her lungs. But nobody knew that.

My mom was fat. And not just "a little overweight." She was fat. She was 5'1" and her weight generally hovered somewhere around 280 pounds. She wore between a size 26 and a 30, depending on the usual vagaries of style, cut, maker, and so forth. She'd been fat for most of my life; I never really knew her as being any different. It was hard for her—her brothers and sisters all take after a different part of the family, so they're all slim and have little trouble staying that way. Where my aunts and uncles are slender-to-trim, my mom was built like an Italian matriarch. She took after their grandmother, who really was an Italian matriarch, and well . . . there you go. Mom became "chubby" in high school, and only got heavier after each of her two pregnancies, and even heavier as she got older and her metabolism slid firmly into neutral. I think she looked at her siblings and felt . . . unfit. Not as in "out of shape," but as in "defective, inadequate, unsatisfactory."

My mom was the kind of person who really, truly believed that if she only followed the rules, she would be rewarded. She would get what she wanted and needed. She just had to follow the rules.

Except, like most people, she had a hard time following the rules. So, while she couldn't follow the rule that said she had to be thin, she did the next best thing and was deeply ashamed of herself and her body. She carried that shame with her everywhere. She tried to not let it slow her down, but there were times when it did. There were times when I think she'd managed to somehow forget she was fat and would try to just live her life, only to get smacked down by some random occurrence that served to put her back in her "place."

Still though, she believed that if she followed the rules, she'd be okay. She avoided having her picture taken. She struggled to remember to wear dark solid-colored clothing, even though she really loved fashion and bright colors and, oh-my-god, the zigzagged sequin-top dress she loved *so much*. Even when we were hip-deep in the eighties and that kind of thing was okay, I thought it was hideous. She loved it. She made a show of not caring how I wrinkled my nose at her when she put it on and wore it anyway. I think though, looking back, that it probably did hurt her feelings a little bit.

My mom was a person whose feelings were always right on the surface. All that shame she carried around about being fat, about having gotten pregnant before she'd gotten married, about every single rule she'd ever broken, every little thing she'd ever thought she'd done "wrong"—it all meant that you didn't have to try very hard to hurt her feelings. They were right there, exposed, and all it took was a word or a sigh or a good eye-roll (and I was a World Champion Eye-Roller by age ten, I tell you what), and she'd be hurt.

And with all that shame, and with so little support from her family or her husband, once my mom got hurt, she had a hard time healing from it.

So when I was about eleven years old, and my mom went to see her doctor because of some problem she was having, and he scathingly told her that her problem was that she was fat and not to come back to him until she'd lost fifty pounds? Yeah. It hurt her. It hurt her bad. But she believed in the rules. And so she tried to ignore how hurt she was and focused on trying extra-hard to get back to following those rules.

She joined Weight Watchers. This was back when you had to buy a little food scale and weigh out your half cups of cottage cheese and three ounces of a boneless, skinless boiled chicken breast or whatever atrocities they made people perpetrate on themselves back then. She tried. She really did try. But she had an eye-rolling eleven-year-old and a whiny seven-year-old and a husband who didn't care what she did, but by God her diet wasn't going to mean he had to eat "that shit," too. He wanted his meat-and-potatoes meals just like always, and if she wanted to cook a separate meal for herself that was fine, but it better not cost much more money than they were already spending on that damn Weight Watchers crap as it was.

After a few months with very limited success, of course she quit. But I tell ya, that goddamn Weight Watchers food scale sat on our kitchen counter for years afterward, almost like some kind of holy relic. Or perhaps it was supposed to be proof to anyone who came over that she really had tried. She really had made the attempt. It was almost like some kind of exhibit, a way to show she was properly ashamed of her fat.

Meanwhile, having been unable to meet her doctor's demand that she lose fifty pounds, she followed the only part of his stated rule that she could: She didn't go back. From that point on, whenever she got sick or injured and someone suggested she go see a doctor, she brushed them off. "Oh, they're just going to tell me I'm too fat. Don't worry, it's just a cold/a sprain/a whatever. I'll be fine."

To be fair, that's not to say she *never* went back again. She did. But only when she had to. And by "had to" I mean she only went when enough people had gotten on her case about whatever it was that she could no longer fend them off with excuses, and she wound up going just to get them off her back. And once my sister and I grew up and left home and my parents divorced, most of us didn't see her frequently enough to strong-arm her into going to the doctor anymore.

It still happened once in a while, which is how she wound up with that asthma inhaler that hardly ever worked. She'd wound up short of breath and wheezing one too many times with my sister around, and finally my sister ordered my mom to see her doctor. So she made the appointment and went, but she took all of her fat-shame with her, and did her best to at least mitigate the awfulness of her sin—that she hadn't lost fifty pounds, and in fact she had gained some more besides: She tried not to take too much of their time. Went in with a probable diagnosis at the ready, even, thanks to her daughters' histories of asthma. She didn't want to bother them too much, you see, even though by then it had been two decades since her last physical. She thanked the doctor when she got the prescription for the inhaler, and never called back when it sometimes didn't work, because she didn't want to take up their valuable time on a rule-breaker like her.

Meanwhile, since the inhaler wasn't working so well, she started to curtail her activities. The adult singles group she was a part of held dances on a regular basis that she'd always been very fond of. She didn't stop going, but she spent most of them sitting on the sidelines or taking pictures. She started to beg off from doing things with my sister and her kids (I had long since moved out of the state), or if she did go along with them to the zoo, she often had to go home early or take frequent breaks. During her last year of life, my mom had given up most of the healthy physical activities she had enjoyed, because her "asthma" was so bad. I'm sure some of those attacks were indeed asthma, but other times she'd wind up out of breath from doing hardly anything at all, and I know it mystified all of us.

A few days before she died, she fell down in a parking lot. Tripped, I guess. The coroner said that may have been what dislodged the blood clot that eventually killed her. Of course, if she'd been getting decent medical care, she might have gotten proper treatment for all of this long before, and maybe she'd still be alive today.

But, you know, that doctor had told her not to come back until she'd lost fifty pounds, and she trusted him. She took him to heart. He was a doctor, after all.

I hope he's proud of himself. His words, more than twenty years ago, helped kill my mother. She spent her last two days in pain, having difficulty breathing, and not once did she call a doctor or try to get some help.

You see, she still hadn't lost those fifty pounds.

CHAPTER SEVEN

Don't Obsess if You Miss
a Day at the Gym

So, you've found a form of exercise you like. And, because it is fun, you're doing it on a regular basis. Maybe you're bopping on down to the gym for water aerobics every Tuesday and Thursday, or you're walking with friends every Wednesday afternoon. Maybe you're going out salsa dancing every Friday night.

But then it happens. Something Comes Up. Because something always comes up. Maybe you have to work late, maybe your kid is sick. Maybe you've injured yourself or you just don't feel good. And you miss a night.

Now there are two options. Option 1 is really common. It's to start freaking out on the roller coaster of guilt. Oh, man, you missed a night of dancing, and now all of your hard work has been for nothing, and you're lazy and bad and worthless.

Except, you're doing this for fun, remember? Which leads to Option 2. This is where you shrug and are sad that you missed the fun of Aquafit but you realize that sometimes things happen, and your nonattendance has nothing to do with your worth as a person. It is no great statement on your discipline or inability to prioritize. It is just a class. Or three.

Sometimes lots of things come up, and you find yourself struggling to stay above water. Is it natural for other activities to take a backseat to making sure the bills are paid and that no one has set the house on fire this week? You betcha.

The problem, the reason that so many women go for Option 1, is that, in our culture, being fit is supposed to be a priority on par with keeping the household from exploding. (Kate has a whole other rant on that being a top priority, but she'll politely refrain just now.) Our social value as women is determined by our looks! How can we maintain our looks if we're too busy making art or spending time with our kids one night to go work out? How? How can we do it all?

We can start by taking a deep breath and remembering something very important. You are exercising because it is fun. (You read that chapter, remember?) It isn't a punishment, and it isn't how you earn your worth as a person. You are exercising because it makes you feel good; making yourself feel horrible about missing a night is deeply counterproductive.

EVERYTHING A LITTLE BIT

There's an all-or-nothing attitude that a lot of women take toward fitness and health. We can view it when it comes to food, and we can view it when it comes to exercise. How many times, while on a diet, did you tell yourself, "Aw, hell, I've had a doughnut for breakfast, the day is shot. Might as well eat all the crap I want today"?

Now, if you're following an intuitive eating plan, you know that you can eat all the crap you want on any day. You can also eat all of the veggies and meat and whatever else that you want. But when you're on a diet and self-denial is a way of living, that one "mistake" is often the signal to give up entirely on your food plan. Same deal with exercise.

This all-or-nothing attitude is unhelpful when it comes to exercise, as well as being the road to self-sabotage when it comes to dieting (which is fine on the one hand, since we fully believe in sabotaging diets, but back before we admitted that dieting was a sucker bet, it wasn't cool). Missing one spinning class—or a month of spinning classes—does not mean you have undone all of the fun and fitness you got from previous classes. It doesn't mean that you've put in a bunch of effort for nothing, because you might have to relearn some things when you go back. The class will be just as fun and you'll still be increasing your fitness.

And if you're just starting out toward a more active lifestyle, remember that any sort of movement is great. You don't have to start running triathlons your first week. So what if you can't keep up with the aerobics instructor? She teaches this class four times a day, three days a week! Remind yourself that exercise is not supposed to be a painful punishment. You'll probably have to remind yourself of this a lot, so it's good to get into the habit in the beginning.

WHEN YOU AREN'T AT THE GYM

It might be a revolutionary thought for some people, but you don't have to go to the gym for a class or to use the weight machines in order to get some exercise. We have this idea in our heads that if it isn't "official" then it doesn't count. Which is, of course, absolutely ridiculous—not to mention classist. A lot of the studies that claim the sky is falling because Americans are so shamefully sedentary are only measuring leisure-time exercises, leaving out a whole lot of people who get more than enough exercise on the job and, P.S., don't have any freakin' leisure time. If you haul baggage or clean houses or move furniture for a living, you're probably (A) plenty fit and (B) not about to hit the gym when you come home exhausted, duh. And even if your job isn't so blatantly physical, chances are, you're not quite as much of a lump as you think. Do you bike to the grocery store? Live in a third-floor walk-up? Mow the lawn? Garden for hours? Have hot sex three times a week? Then you are already doing something that increases fitness; you are not just lying around on the couch all the time, even if that's how you think of your activity level.

Similarly, an important part of learning to exercise for pleasure rather than weight loss or self-torture is getting over the idea that if it's fun, it can't possibly count. For example, Marianne likes to go dancing. At one point, during the grand college days of her youth, Marianne was going dancing five nights a week. She wasn't sleeping or eating, but, hey, she was having a good time. But when people asked her if she was exercising, her answer was always no.

A night out dancing meant four or five hours of actual dancing, accompanied by five or six bottles of water. It meant Marianne's heart rate was elevated and all of her muscles were involved in keeping her from falling down. She came home sweaty and exhausted, but also exhilarated from the constant movement. But for some reason, despite all of the exercise going on, it just didn't count. Maybe because there was loud music and a lot of other people and no gym clothes. Maybe because it didn't feel like a punishment for being fat. Who knows? But Marianne didn't give herself credit for all of that activity until a couple of years later when a personal trainer, of all people, lectured her about how not all exercise had to come from the gym.

If you take your dog for long walks, you are getting exercise. If you live in New York City and climb the stairs from the subway every day, you are getting exercise. If you chase a toddler around your backyard, you are getting a ton of exercise! Will these things lead to optimum fitness? Well, it depends on the dog and the station and the toddler, but probably not. Doesn't matter. The point is, you're already a basically active person, so adding some more activity shouldn't be this hugely daunting thing. Give yourself a little credit for what you're already doing.

THE BIG REVEAL

"Okay, but get back to the skipping the gym thing!" we hear you saying. "What happens if that night or two I've missed turns into six months?"

Here's the big secret: Nothing. Nothing happens. You don't turn into a bad person. You don't have to mentally castigate yourself or ask other people to shame you into going back. We'd suggest figuring out why you haven't gone back, though, if it is really bothering you. Why did it stop being fun? And if it just isn't fun anymore, then it's time to try something else. Fitness monogamy is not required.

Know why? *You're exercising because it's fun.* Remember that. If you're having fun, you won't have to force yourself to go back. And if you do have to force yourself because it just isn't fun, you need to go back to the drawing board and find a form of exercise that is.

CHAPTER EIGHT

Don't Weigh Yourself

The scale. It sits there, waiting to judge you, a flat little square (or rectangle or whatever) of horror. It's a tyrant, demanding you take off your shoes first, or your weight will be elevated (because shoes can weigh twenty extra pounds, you know), demanding that you don't weigh yourself in the morning (because you are bloated), demanding that you care what it has to tell you. It's such a small thing to have such ridiculous power over women.

Marianne hasn't owned a scale in years. But that didn't stop her from weighing herself every single day at the gym during the height of her numbers obsession. And then, even after she had started working on not caring about the number on the scale, she joined Curves, with its weekly measurements and weigh-in, and that got her all wound up back in the emotional tangle of the numbers. (Note: Kate has also worked out at Curves in the past and did not have to submit to any such thing—this probably varies by location.) The same thing happened at Weight Watchers.

And, with the knot of obsession firmly planted in her belly (which was not shrinking on any of these programs), everything she did became about making the numbers move. Activities stopped being about fun and feeling good. They became solely about losing weight. And when she couldn't lose weight, no matter what she tried, all of the other health benefits she enjoyed from being active stopped mattering. Luckily, Marianne wised up. She knows her weight, because being weighed at the doctor's office is no longer a traumatic experience, and it helps her doctor figure out dosages for allergy medications. But the important thing is, she doesn't care what the number is anymore.

THE INSANITY OF NUMBERS

If you are at all a collector of data or analytically minded or the tiniest bit compulsive, it is amazingly easy to fall into the power of the scale. It provides a concrete number. It should be a neutral value. But it becomes a measure of "progress"—when the number is going down—or a measure of backsliding—when the number is going up—when you are dieting and substituting weight loss for health.

That's the source of the scale's power; we think it will tell us something fundamental about ourselves. It will reveal our depth of commitment to weight loss, to improving ourselves, to being the best we can be.

But, y'all, the best we can be is not exclusively determined by physical measures. The best we can be is highly subjective and may, according to your personal definition, have more to do with how well you treat other people or how well you use your skills and talents. Unless you are a jockey or a boxer, knowing what you weigh down to the pound really has very little connection to achieving what you want in life.

In fact, obsessing about that number leads to madness. We had one reader of the blogs mention that she bought herself a digital scale to keep track of fractions of pounds lost, weight that wouldn't register on a regular scale. She was excited every time she lost two-tenths of a pound and angry when she gained two-tenths. That is giving way too much crazy power to the scale and the number on it.

The number on the scale is actually pretty irrelevant as a measure of health. If you are practicing Health At Every Size, then you already know that defining health is a personal endeavor. Instead, of checking your weight, check out your numbers for blood sugar and blood pressure and cholesterol and triglycerides.

If your numbers are right smack where they are supposed to be and you have not magically become thin, understand that this is not a miraculous occurrence that has happened in spite of your fat. If those numbers aren't where your doctor thinks they should be, it may have nothing to do with your fat. It may have to do with your eating or exercise habits, but if you've read this far, you know those things are separate from what you weigh. We know it is easy to blame that stuff on your body for being larger than some arbitrary number on a chart thinks it should be—especially if your doctor is feeding you that same line—but don't fall for it. Find a new doctor, one who treats you with respect, and ask around in your family. If they have a history of high blood pressure, why would you expect to dodge that bullet?

Lots of health issues have a strong genetic component. We're not advocating that you throw your hands up in the air and abandon all hope because your great-grandmother had heart disease, but we are saying that you don't have to blame your fat and hate yourself because of it. Instead, focus on improving your fitness levels and making sure your diet isn't too lopsided. Beating yourself up and trying to lose weight isn't going to solve anything and may actually make the problem worse—remember back in Chapter 1 when we talked about the negative health impacts of dieting? Staying off the scale will keep you focused on doing good things for your heart instead of focused on your weight.

Also keep in mind that your weight is going to fluctuate a bit no matter what you are eating and doing. It's the nature of bodies; they are not static things but are living organisms with a bunch of unseen processes always taking place. That means sometimes—and anyone who has ever been on their period should know this—your body is going to retain water. That is going to affect your weight. If you weigh yourself before and after going to the bathroom, not to gross anyone out, your weight will show the effects! (Especially if you've got a digital scale.) This is normal. You cannot control every fluctuation in weight. Trying will just lead to tears and, possibly, self-destructive behaviors because you think you aren't being "good" enough.

It is entirely possible that your doctor needs to know your weight for calculating dosages. If that isn't true, though, you don't even have to be weighed at the doctor's office. Tell your doctor ahead of time, and don't let the nurse drag you over to the scale automatically. If they insist, let them know you don't want to know the number—turn around and don't look while they weigh you. Unless you've had a rapid, unexplained weight gain or loss—in which case, you really should look into a possible medical reason for it—your weight shouldn't be a primary topic of discussion at the doctor's office.

The scale in your bathroom or bedroom? Throw it out. Don't let that petty tyrant continue to rule you. Do your jeans still fit (even when they are fresh out of the dryer)? Then your weight is about the same as it was yesterday. And, really, that's all any of us need to know.

PART THREE

{ socializing }

CHAPTER NINE

Find a Good Partner

Sad but true: Most of the people we see writing confidently and persuasively about body acceptance in general and fat acceptance specifically are married or in solid long-term relationships. There aren't nearly as many single people doing this, as far as we can tell. And that is kind of heartbreaking, because we suspect that it is no mere coincidence.

It's really hard to stand up to the constant barrage of anti-fat messages, the incessant refrains of "Fat is hideously unattractive" and "Who could love a fat person?" when you don't have the concrete reminder of a partner's presence that you are both attractive and lovable. And if you're searching for a partner, it can be twice as hard, because you have no real control over changing your single status. Sure, you can do all the things the magazines tell you—going out to parties or bars, cultivating hobbies that involve other people, placing an online personal ad, and so on—but, at the end of the day, there is a certain element of luck to finding a partner. A pretty darn big element of luck, in fact.

When you're single, it's all too easy to spend your time looking for reasons why. Why is this happening to you? Why are you still alone? And all the people trying to sell you shit are happy to provide answers: It's because your teeth aren't white enough, your skin isn't smooth and clear, your hair is the wrong color, you smell funny, you're not wearing the right bra. (You probably aren't wearing the right bra, but that's not why you're single.) And oh yeah, it's because you're too fat. Even if you're thin.

If you can just fix everything that is wrong with you, the story goes—even if the fixes are just illusions attained with a push-up bra and some Spanx—you can have your pick of partners, your life will be perfect, you'll achieve happiness and companionship without even trying. An invisible gate will open, allowing all those people you always knew would love you if you were just a little prettier to walk right through and ask what you're doing Friday night. Manufacturers and ad agencies are trying to sell you this idea—what Kate calls the Fantasy of Being Thin—because it makes them a lot of money. People who like their bodies and know that "single" isn't synonymous with "unlovable" don't tend to buy a lot of cellulite cream.

And, consciously, you know that. We all know this is bullshit. We look at the Tummy Tamer panel in the swimsuit and know that it is not going to transform us into a flat-bellied movie star. We know that any relationship based solely on looks is going to be a shallow thing, and at some point we'll have to take off our makeup masks of perfection. We know all of this, but sometimes the notion that being single is our own fault—as if it were a punishment from some higher authority—still gets its hooks into us.

So, we get it. We've been through it, and, even though we're both in good relationships, we remember with more than a little twinge the unhappy feeling of having no one to call when we've had a Really Bad Day, no one who would bring us Chinese food and watch our favorite movies and take care of us until we felt better. And we know how much freakin' luck is involved in finding that person—which means that when we suggest getting yourself a good partner as a step toward loving your body (and yourself!), we know this one is a real doozy. But, please, hear us out. We promise we aren't going to repeat the same old crap about how you have to love yourself before someone will love you. There are plenty of screamingly insecure married people out there already, you know?

THE FIRST RULE OF FAT CLUB

Here is the one simple rule we want you to take from this chapter: You are not allowed to settle for someone who is not totally crazy about you and your naked body. That means no settling for a secret relationship with a guy who wants to fuck you but not introduce you to his friends. No getting serious with a woman who says she wants what is best for you but constantly belittles your chub. No hanging on to the dude who judgmentally pokes your belly fat or the girl who monitors your caloric intake. Those kinds of people? Not good partners.

A good partner is someone who loves you for who you are, not for who he or she wants you to become. That means they love you when you are dressed to the nines and also when you've just rolled out of bed and are wondering if bunny slippers count toward the No Shirt, No Shoes, No Service rule at your local grocery store. It means they respect your intelligence, your opinions, your body autonomy, and can disagree with you without attacking who you are as a person—meaning they don't get to call you a fat cow when they're mad and then expect you to brush it off.

Of course, the obvious question now is, even if you can't totally control the outcome, how can you go about looking for a good partner? Fortunately, we've done some legwork so you don't have to.

THE SETUP

First, let your friends know you're looking. We know, we know, blind dates and matchmaking are utterly passé. But if your friends know you well, then they might actually have some insight when it comes to the type of person you'd enjoy dating. Kate was dating up a storm, doing pretty well in terms of quantity if not quality, when her friend Paula introduced her to this guy named Al—while she was on a date with someone else, in fact. (It was a group outing.) Paula didn't mention she thought Kate and Al would be great together, though she secretly did— she just put them in a room together and let them figure it out. As it turned out, she was a way better judge of Kate's tastes than

Kate was; the date she'd brought was an unbelievable drag, but Al was damn near love at first sight. He moved in with her three months later and didn't appear to be going anywhere when this book went to press, two and a half years after that. Marianne's friends weren't even that subtle when they set her up with the cute guy she wound up marrying. They just kept sending her evidence of how cute he was until she expressed some interest.

This is not to say you should trust any old friend to pair you off, of course. Here's Marianne's rule of thumb: If you don't trust them to pick out a movie for you, they probably aren't going to pick out a great date for you either. You do not have to rush right out when your mom tells you about the new cashier at her local supermarket or Betty's son the doctor or the nice young man down the street. "He's single!" does not constitute sufficient grounds for assuming compatibility, no matter what she says. But as with job hunting, networking never hurts, and you never know who's going to have the right lead. Let your friends know you're in the market.

DON'T WAIT FOR A DATE

Second, continue to live your life. As hard as it can be to believe—and we know it can be really hard to believe—there is nothing wrong with you being single. It might not be ideal, but it isn't the end of your life. Go about the business of being yourself and working to improve your life in other ways. This is important for a couple of reasons. One, if you aren't going to sit around putting off your life until you are thin (and you aren't, right?), why would you put off starting your life until you are partnered? Two, self-confidence and having a full and interesting life are attractive qualities in a person. Would you want to be with someone who wasn't doing anything at all with their life except waiting around for you to show up? (Hint: The answer is no.) So go out and do all the things you want to do. Go to school, learn new skills, take up tennis, travel, all of that stuff. If you won't do it because you believe you deserve to have fun while you're single, then do it because that might be how you meet The One.

YOU HAVE TO BE FINDABLE

Next, put yourself out there. This is a little more active than just telling your friends that you are available. This means all of that scary stuff like Internet personal ads, speed dating, and trolling the dog park. (Kate has actually done all of those things, so we're not just talking out our asses here.) Even more frighteningly, if you're fat, it also means telling people you meet online or through personals that you're fat, and posting or sending a picture before you meet in person.

We won't shit you; unless you're on a BBW site, that will probably get you less traffic than only posting a head shot taken at a double-chin-concealing angle. But that's less traffic from people who don't want to date fat women, not from potential dream partners. Having a drawn-out email flirtation with someone who has no idea what you look like will almost never lead to that person falling so madly in love with your mind, your looks will be irrelevant. Much more often, it will lead to the person being angry you withheld that information—which is relevant, as it happens. Aren't looks relevant to you? You may not have a particular type, and you may be strongly attracted to people who deviate from the cultural beauty standards, but there are still some people you find unattractive, for whatever reason, right? Does that mean you're a shallow asshole if you don't want to date those people? No. You're just an individual with individual tastes. And so is any person who happens to find you unattractive—even if we all are, of course, influenced by a kabillion sources telling us only thin women can be beautiful.

The fact is, not everyone's drunk the Beauty Myth Kool-Aid, and those who have aren't people you want to go out with anyway, so forget them. That girl who stopped writing back when she saw your picture might be a shallow asshole, or she might just have bad memories of an ex who's practically your doppelgänger. Who knows? Who cares? If someone doesn't think you're hot, you do not want to date that person, period. And you definitely don't want to try to trick someone into finding you attractive. Putting yourself out there means putting yourself out there—not some disembodied version of you that the dude you're chatting with can layer over his vision of a supermodel. It means owning your body just as much as your mind and believing that if someone doesn't like your body, that person isn't right for you. You are not a brain in a jar, for Pete's sake; your body is you. If someone doesn't want it, then she doesn't want you. And if someone doesn't want you, then it follows that you don't want him or her—get it?

Of course, no matter how much you believe that, rejection still sucks. We aren't gonna lie about it. You answer the personal ad of someone you think is interesting, and they send back a thanks but no thanks—or, worse, never even respond at all—and it sucks. It's hard not to take that personally, because, well, it is personal. But it helped Marianne, when she was dealing with rejection, to remember that things like this are always just as much about the other person as they were about her. Kate's greatest piece of advice is to remember that the rejection could be about any number of things, not just the things you don't like about yourself and thus assume other people won't like about you. Marianne could have told herself some guy didn't write back because she was fat, when for all she knew, he thought she was gorgeous but didn't write back because her profile said she loved *Star Trek*. (And why would she want to be with a dude who didn't love *Star Trek*?!) Kate could have told herself a guy bolted in abject fear of her thighs, when he was actually turned off by her intractable potty mouth. And either of us could have fallen victim to an email trapped in a spam filter, a family emergency, another cute fat woman who came along just moments before and stole the guy's heart—a zillion different reasons for perceived rejection that actually had nothing at all to do with us.

Unless someone actually takes the time to write back and say, "NO THX UR UGLY" (and hey, it's the Internet, so we have to admit that could happen), you have absolutely no idea why they rejected you. So instead of sitting around cataloguing all your flaws, trying to put your finger on precisely which repulsive attribute of yours caused the blow off, why not assume it wasn't about you? Trust us, indulging in a maudlin fit of self-flagellation will not actually yield any important insights about your singleness.

Here's the thing: You are exactly what someone is looking for, and that someone is exactly what you are looking for, too. You don't have to be prettier. You don't have to be thinner. You just have to be you—even if you're a fat girl wearing sweatpants, with uncombed hair and no makeup (as the authors of this book are much of the time). The problem is not you; it's just that you don't know when or where you're going to run into that person, so you can't do a damned thing to speed up the process. For as much as Western culture insists hard work will get you everything you want—and the speed at which your desires are met will be directly proportional to the amount of effort you put out—it just doesn't work that way all the time. Your mama was right: Life isn't fair. If it were, we'd all be in love right now, because we all deserve it, right now. There are very few people in this world who actually don't deserve love. (Marianne might be enough of a hippy to say there are no people who don't deserve love, but Kate will at least make an exception for sociopaths, who wouldn't appreciate it anyway.)

If you're not in a relationship right now, it's not because you're too plain or too fat or because you snort when you laugh or your shampoo smells like the wrong kind of flowers. It's just because you haven't yet bumped into someone who digs you the most and vice versa. If you had to be tall, thin, clear-skinned, straight-haired, and so on to be worthy of love, Marianne wouldn't be ecstatically married (which is a phrase she never imagined herself using), and Kate wouldn't be happily living with her partner. The idea that conventional beauty is a prerequisite for being loved and desired is a big freakin' lie. Unfortunately, it's a lie that will be with us as long as insecurity and low self-esteem keep driving women to whip out their credit cards. If we all believed we deserved love just as we are, the economy would probably grind to a halt.

Which brings us back to the point of the chapter. We'll even restate it in different words. Do not settle for anyone less than a good partner who is crazy about you. You deserve better, and you know better.

Relationships are work, obviously, but no one is paying you to put up with a shitty one. Being alone is better than being in a bad relationship—which can wreck your self-confidence even faster than the latest issue of *Cosmo*. Wait for someone who sees beauty in your body as well as your mind, even if you can't see it yet. (That's what the rest of this book is for.)

CHAPTER TEN

Stop Judging Other Women

Her roots are three inches long. Her gut makes her look pregnant. Her ass has its own ZIP code. Who told her that top goes with that skirt? She is SO much fatter than I am.

It's like a litany in our heads whenever we're out in public, surrounded by other women, or even just watching them on TV: a constant stream of judgment that assigns ranks to every woman we see, as though we'll be lost unless we know our place. At some point in your adult life, you've probably walked into a party and felt a frisson of relief upon discovering at least one woman there who was fatter, uglier, and/or dressed more inappropriately than you. We sure have. But if you want to have any hope of making peace with your own body, you need to knock that shit off.

We're not even telling you to stop just because it's nasty, petty, and beneath you to judge other women so harshly; it is, but you're not a saint, and neither are we. We're telling you to stop because it's actually in your own self-interest to stop being such a bitch. 'Cause you know what happens when you quit saying that crap about other women? You magically stop saying it about yourself so much, too.

Judging other women negatively creates a constant stream of nasty thoughts in your head. It is inevitable that you will end up applying those same standards to yourself. We think we're building ourselves up when we do this but, really, we're just tearing other people down to our level. And we hate to go all Mr. Rogers' Neighborhood on you, but tearing other people down isn't really productive. It leaves you in the same place you started, which is full of loathing for your own body.

EVEN SKINNY WOMEN GET THE BODY BLUES

Sadly, when you're in that place, you're far from alone. According to the National Eating Disorders Association's website, different surveys have shown that 42 percent of first to third grade girls want to be thinner, 81 percent of ten-year-olds are afraid of being fat, and 91 percent of college-aged women have attempted to lose weight.[1] The (Canadian) National Eating Disorder Information Centre's website reports that 80 to 90 percent of grown women dislike the size and shape of their bodies.[2] Among five thousand women surveyed by the British magazine NW in 2007, 84 percent said they would be happier if they could lose weight.[3] We wish we could say we're shocked by those numbers, but we're not. We live in a culture in which women are constantly picked apart by viewers of all sorts. From the media to family members to strangers, there is always an audience looking at women to see if they measure up to whatever ideal is being presented as fashionable at any given time.

We are held to a standard that can only be achieved by a tiny handful of real, live women. (Remember the old Body Shop ad that said, "There are 3 billion women in the world who don't look like supermodels, and only 8 who do"? We loved that ad.) And even the women who do meet the beauty standard aren't presented to us as they really look. Thanks to Photoshop, those impossibly beautiful women really are impossibly beautiful— when you see them in magazines, they've had inches shaved off their thighs and arms, their necks lengthened, their laugh lines removed, their boobs elevated, their eyes enlarged, and on and on. Even the models don't look like their own pictures. So why are we judging ourselves by these impossible standards? Why are we judging other women by them, too?

FEAR AND LOATHING

Marianne is a people watcher. She likes sitting in a location and observing the parade that inevitably passes by. But, at a club she used to go to with a bunch of friends, this turned into a concentrated critique of every woman (and most of the men) in the room. Was it funny? Sure, at the time (she was eighteen). Was it potentially hurtful to other people? Yes, if they had heard. Was it in any way useful? Not at all. Because by nitpicking the appearance of other people, Marianne more fully trained herself to nitpick her OWN appearance. If she was willing to make fun of someone else's crooked eyeliner, well, her own crooked eyeliner was even more unacceptable. After all, it might give someone else reason to make fun of her.

That fear settled in as well. If Marianne were sitting around judging other people, certainly other people were sitting around judging her! And that was a frightening thought. It wound up making her more and more self-conscious. It made getting ready to go out to that particular club an exercise in anxiety and self-loathing instead of, you know, an exercise in picking out fancy dancing pants. And so Marianne realized she had to stop. Because snarking on other people's clothing choices was doing a lot more harm than good.

If judging other women's clothing choices did that much harm, how much more harmful would judging other women's bodies have been? Exponentially more harmful. Clothing is, in large part, a choice that is consciously made. Our bodies are a much larger part of our identities than our wardrobes are, and they are much harder (if not impossible) to change. Get into the habit of hating other women's bellies, and your own belly will start to look worse and worse. Get into the habit of looking to see who has less than perfectly toned arms, and your own will quickly grow annoyingly flappy in your mind—without changing a bit in reality.

In contrast, when Marianne started looking at other people with kindness (a habit she has continued to cultivate through the years), when she started consciously looking for the good things about other people, it was a lot easier to see those good things in herself.

And maybe it really is that simple (though forming the habit takes some effort)—we see what we expect to see. If we're looking for flaws, for faults, and other weaknesses we can use to create a hierarchy of attractiveness, that is what we are going to see when we look at others and when we look at ourselves. If we're looking for beauty, it's going to be everywhere, in everyone, including ourselves.

Wow, that was sappy. We promise to be less feel-good in the next chapter.

Fatness and Uplift
Not an Essay About Push-Up Bras

by Julia Starkey

The way I primarily self-identify is as someone who is mixed race (black and Swedish). I talk about being black in this essay, because that is an identity I also inhabit. I don't "look mixed" or like I have passing privilege. When it comes to societal expectations and race, I'm black.

Although this essay focuses on my being a fat woman of color, I'm going to begin by talking about my dad. My father's way of thinking about life was deeply influenced by W.E.B. DuBois and ideas of racial uplift and the talented tenth. His parents were part of the Great Migration and ended up in Indianapolis. His grandfather had fled Georgia with a heavily pregnant wife, because of an altercation with a white man in town. When my father's parents bought their house, they were the first black family to own in the neighborhood (only semi-legally, since the deed to the house specified it could not be sold to Negroes). My father's parents emphasized education as the path to freedom. Their views were part of a general belief in racial uplift. By working hard, educating oneself, and generally setting a good example to other black people, we would help all of us get ahead.

Racial uplift wasn't just about educated black elites giving other black people a helping hand; it was also about showing white people that blacks were not a collection of negative stereotypes. The people at the forefront (the talented tenth) had to be smart, neat, clean, articulate, and, above all, they couldn't get angry about racism. Instead, dressed in your best suit, you presented carefully constructed arguments against racism, knowing that any misstep would be taken as proof that blacks really were inferior.

Presenting oneself well, in the best suit, was an important aspect of being the stereotype breakers. In order to have a chance of being taken seriously, you had to look clean and put together from head to foot. Your hair had to be neat (and for women carefully straightened) because frizzy hair made you look like a "bush person." The best way to describe the look is "controlled." If negative stereotypes about black people were about them being savage, flighty, ruled by emotion, and lacking reasoning, then the way to counter that was to look modern, tailored, and never have a hair out of place.

When I think about how this applies to me, I look to my father's mother and his sisters, all of whom are fat black women. My grandmother died when I was young, so my memories of her aren't very clear. But in photographs of her, she is always carefully and neatly dressed with handbags that matched her outfits. Even when she had to ride the bus for more than two hours to get to the office she worked at, she always dressed carefully. No one could accuse of her being sloppy or lazy, and the same for her children. Her daughters, my aunts, dress more casually, but with an emphasis on looking "pulled together." Their clothes always fit nicely, their hair is neat, and nothing is scuffed or worn out. One of my aunts has cancer, and even though she is dealing with chemo, she is still putting together stylish outfits. When she was visiting my family she came down to breakfast wearing silk PJs with an abstract gold print and a cocoa-colored silk wrap and had wrapped a purple silk scarf attractively around her head.

Being concerned about looking "presentable" is an issue many people face, but it has particular relevance for fat black women. The image that we are fighting back against is the popular—and powerful—image of black women as mammies.

Mammies are fat and happy all the time. Mammies have dark, shiny/greasy skin, rolling white eyes, gleaming white teeth, and a kerchief tied over unruly hair. Mammies are never attractive, and they are also desexualized. Mammies just love to engage in menial labor for white people. Mammies are humble and grateful for what they have and don't think of overreaching themselves to do better. Mammies don't want to rock the boat. Mammies are the opposite of what those seeking to better themselves want to be.

Because mammy figures are such a potent image, fat black women have to put in extra effort to not fit into the stereotype. This is why my aunts always paid careful attention to what they wore to work, erring toward professional rather than casual. Why they have steadfastly gone after promotions. Why they joined service organizations to help their communities. This is why they would never dream of leaving the house with a kerchief wrapped around their heads (the silk scarf my aunt knotted around her head was too elegant to be called a kerchief, and besides she was with family). I'll run to the corner store in PJs, but you'll never see me with a red kerchief wrapped around my head.

I'm my father's daughter, and he raised me with these ideas of uplift and doing better both for myself as an individual, but also as a member of the black community. It's one of those things that was never explicitly discussed in my home but pervaded everything. In the suburbs where I grew up, my father was the only black adult in the area. It wasn't until I was in eighth grade that there was another black student in my grade. Despite the lack of other physical black bodies, the presence of the stereotypes was always there. For better or worse, I mostly got "you're not like those black people" or "I don't think of you as black," which, well . . . I was too young to really know how to respond to the racism embedded in both of those statements. I was succeeding in not being a stereotype, but instead of breaking down stereotypes about black people, my background ended up being erased.

It was in college that the importance of having an appropriately positive body really came home for me. I went to an ivy league school. Contrary to what people think about the school, the black community around me wasn't just rich black elites: Plenty of us were on financial aid with significant student loans. We were united in the belief that we could better ourselves through education.

The other thing that united the black students was not looking "ghetto" (and yes, there is internalized prejudice there that I don't want to get into right now). No "extreme" hair, no big jewelry, baggy jeans, exposed curlers, or loud attitudes. And definitely no jiggling flesh on display. Being fat was something you needed to control. Fatness was more often talked about in the context of the endemic problems of diabetes and high blood pressure in the black community, than in a positive affirming way.

Although the black students didn't look like they fell out of a J. Crew catalog, even at breakfast the black students tended to be more pulled together than their white compatriots, so it was clear they weren't the hired help. We disassociated ourselves from anything that would make white students forget we were there to labor with our minds not our bodies. Having a fat body that reminded people of a servant lacing up Scarlett O'Hara didn't fit the cultivated image of the educated elite. We didn't want the white students and faculty around us to forget that we were budding elites, too.

The situation makes me think of Lena Horne's father, who, in the 1950s, said he hired maids for his daughter, and she wasn't going to play one in the movies (with the NAACP's backing, this was written into her film studio contract). This, of course, is in contrast to Hattie McDaniel, who played almost nothing but maids and mammies during her film career. Lena Horne's image as a glamorous, talented, successful black woman was also built on her slim body and pale skin. She was the opposite of a fat, dark mammy figure. Horne's sleek tailored look, and beautifully controlled voice, made her someone the NAACP could stand behind.

It frustrates me when I hear white women in the fat acceptance community talk about how fat-positive the black community is and express bitterness/jealously that "their community" isn't, when they've never talked to a fat black woman about what her experience of fatness is like. The existence of the song "Baby Got Back" or the popularity of Queen Latifah are presented as proof of how fat-accepting black people are. However, those examples are taken from black pop culture white people like and are chosen without looking at the complexities of what fat black female bodies have meant both historically and in the present. "Baby Got Back" is not actually about fat women. It's about women with "an itty bitty waist and a round thing in your face" and who look like Flo-Jo, the Olympic athlete. On a related note, Sir Mix-A-Lot's line, "*Cosmo* ain't got nothin' to do with my selection. 36-24-36? Ha, only if she's 5'3"" is a reference to the 1970s funk song "Brick House," by the Commodores. In "Brick House," the singer rhapsodizes about a big stacked woman; however, her measurements are given as "36-24-36, what a winning hand!" These songs are about women with big boobs and butts and a defined waist, not necessarily someone with an overall large body. If I were going to pick a song that is fat-positive, I'd go with "Sista Big Bones," by Anthony Hamilton. He selected Mo'Nique to be the star of the video.

My experience of being a fat black woman has not been a fat-acceptance wonderland. I don't feel like I have been shamed for my body, but I have felt pressure to have a more socially acceptable body size. I do worry about presenting myself well. Because of the history and attitudes in my community, I feel a responsibility to act in a manner that adheres to a strict code of conduct. Part of the code is hiding its existence from mainstream white culture. I struggle with those pressures when I don't feel like pulling myself together, when I want to toss a scarf over my messy hair and go grab some milk at the store, when I want to snarl at someone rather than do racism 101 for the umpteenth time. Being told by white women that I have it easy when it comes to body image dismisses all of the complexities and difficulties of my identity and reduces them to "*Cosmo* says you're fat. Well, I ain't down with that!"

Making assumptions about someone's identity and culture based on fragments of pop culture is dehumanizing. An important part of understanding the world beyond yourself is not just asking questions, but also listening closely to people who have criticisms of your beliefs. Sometimes what you think is fact is based on false premises. Black women do not live in a fat-acceptance utopia, and you're making racist assumptions if you assume they do.

CHAPTER ELEVEN

Get a Hobby That Has Nothing to Do with Your Weight (And Do It with Other People)

What do you love to do? When you're on your lunch break at work, thinking about the evening ahead, what are your plans? If the only thing you have to look forward to is network television (or, hell, even cable!), it might be time to find a new hobby.

Now, we're not knocking television. There are some great shows on TV and some fantastic stories being told. But the idiot box is a major source of body-hating messages, and by spending hours in front of it, you are just absorbing more lies about how you aren't good enough. Do we really need more of those messages in our lives? Hell, no!

But you're busy, you say, and you're tired. We understand. We feel the same way. Coming home after a long day at work and turning on a favorite show to watch in your comfy pants can be a perfectly delightful activity. We aren't here to deny that to anyone. We're just saying you might already have more potential free time than you realize.

How often do you think about what to eat at your next meal? If you're on a diet, it's pretty often. Planning meals, counting calories, and attending weekly weigh-ins takes more time and energy than you might imagine. Even if you're not actively dieting, the energy you spend feeling guilty about eating the "wrong" things, worrying that you might gain weight, and imagining what you'd do if only you lost weight can be significant. Dieting and self-loathing can become not just hobbies but part-time jobs, if you let them. If you took all of that time and energy and focused it somewhere else, just imagine what you could do! Knitting, dog sledding, building a scale model of the Taj Mahal out of toothpicks and marshmallows . . . the world is your oyster when you are no longer stressing about the size of your ass.

GETTING OUT OF YOUR HEAD

Simple fact: When you are volunteering to serve meals to the homeless, you are too busy to feel guilty about the class you missed at the gym. When you are deep in the midst of a project, there is no room to be thinking about whether or not your hips are in proportion to the rest of your body. No way! You're too busy actually accomplishing something. And in addition to getting you out of your head, hobbies provide a real sense of accomplishment and pride—when those feelings aren't linked to transitory things like weight loss, you actually get to keep them. That's a good thing. Taking real pride and pleasure in the things that you do can boost your confidence in all areas of your life—including with regard to your body. It's hard to feel bad about your body when you are using it to do awesome things, after all.

It's way too easy to start feeling like your body is the root of all your problems, and everyone is staring at you and judging you, when you aren't doing anything that creates a sense of perspective. When your inner world is limited to you and your self-loathing, it is a lot easier to believe that the guy on the bus who smiled at you was really laughing at how fat you are.

MAKING NEW FRIENDS

Getting out and doing things with other people can be a powerful antidote to that kind of destructive self-absorption. Engaging with your community is one terrific way to reinforce that making your thighs smaller isn't first on anyone else's list of things to do; what seems like a huge problem hanging over your head is, in the company of others (provided they're not assholes), revealed to be a total non-issue.

If you're not happy with the friends you've got or would just like to add more to your crew, finding a hobby you love is one way to fix that problem. Sharing a common interest gives you something to talk about with new people, obviously, and doing something together can make conversation flow more easily than it might over coffee with a stranger you found on Craig's List.

Find something you love, something that isn't about your weight, something that you can do alone or with other people. Find something you can feel passionate about, something that moves you to try new things, discover new talents, learn new skills. Find something that pushes you a little bit out of your comfort zone and that's exhilarating because you love what you are able to accomplish. Find that, and we promise, you'll spend a lot less time worrying about the size of your jeans and a lot more time remembering how awesome you can be.

CHAPTER TWELVE

Don't Believe That Only Sick Freaks Would Want to Date Fat Women

Our society's "hot-or-not" arbiters rarely admit that some people date fatties on purpose. And when they do admit it, it's usually with a clear implication that those people must be sick freaks. Those who express interest in fat women are shamed for liking bodies that are outside the mainstream beauty ideal. And women who are fat are told that, because they have failed at being Beautiful, according to this particular culture at this particular time, they're worthless; no one who is any good could ever love them. It's all a huge crock, but after you've heard those messages a couple zillion times, it's hard not to believe them.

Combine these pervasive lies with a bunch of salacious media stories about fetishists and "feeders" (people who are sexually aroused by seeing their partners eat massive amounts of food and/or gain weight*), and you wind up with fat women who think anyone who finds them attractive must have a nasty ulterior motive or be some sort of pervert. Now, for the record, we don't believe that fetishism necessarily equals perversion, but if that isn't your thing—and for a lot of people, including us, it's not—there's no reason why you should have to find someone with a fat fetish or die alone.

WHAT'S YOUR PROBLEM?

There are lots of people, just plain regular folks, who think fat women are beautiful. There are also lots of other people who will think so once they've met the right fat woman. And then there are people known as "fat admirers," who are not interested in force-feeding you or objectifying your body but simply have a natural preference for the look of a fat person, just as other people strongly prefer those who are muscular or tall or, yes, thin. Some fat admirers describe it as more of a sexual orientation than a mere preference—they're only attracted to fat people, and have

---

*A word of caution: Fat fetishists may simply be individuals who require fat partners to reach sexual fulfillment. But feederism, a fetish that involves feeding a partner with the explicit goal of their gaining large amounts of weight, is a bit different. Generally speaking, we don't advise hooking up with anyone who wants you to change your body—whether that means losing weight or gaining it—for their sexual gratification. Be open to different possibilities and have a good time, but be smart, too. Remember, you're looking for a good partner, and that means someone who is right for you, not just someone who will settle for you.

known from a young age that they were "different"—but either way, they're sincerely and non-creepily drawn to fat partners. All of these people who actively want to date larger women are not weird or kinky or desperate (though some probably are and hey, weird and kinky can be a lot of fun). They are just people who find fat women attractive, the way other people think redheads are to die for. Some people like girls who wear glasses, and some people like fat girls who wear glasses.

So, where the hell *are* those people? This might sting a little, but we need to give it to you straight. If you rarely meet people who seem like they are (or could be) warm for your form, the problem is probably not your form. The problem is probably stuff that's not much easier, but a lot more satisfying, to change. Like everyone else, fat admirers and other folks who are attracted to fat women are looking for partners who are confident and fun to be around. Here's the plain truth: Nobody's less attractive than people who can't stop obsessing about how unattractive they are.

Kate was single all through college, and the whole time, she blamed it on her body. Never mind that she saw fatter women with partners all over the place. (Those guys were sick freaks, obvy!) And never mind that she was walking around with untreated depression, a permascowl on her face, and the sort of fuck-you attitude that is the hallmark of the middle-class nineteen-year-old who thinks she's already seen the whole world and finds it *so damned boring*. Clearly, she was only unattractive because she was fat!

It took a long time for her to realize that she could have been built like a model, and . . . well, wait, let's be honest. If she'd been built like a model, she probably would have gotten laid more in college. It's college, for Pete's sake. But she wouldn't have gotten laid as much as a model-type with a pleasant personality! And she almost certainly wouldn't have found a good, healthy relationship with a great guy, because great people who are capable of having healthy relationships aren't interested in dating insecure, hateful basket cases.

When you tell yourself that no one could possibly be attracted to you—and carry yourself in a way that reflects that thinking—the message you're sending the world is not, as you probably believe somewhere deep down, "Please, please, someone come along and tell me I'm not as ugly as I think I am!" It's: "What kind of an asshole would be attracted to me? Hey, you there—did you just have a moment where you thought I was pretty? Well, you're *wrong*! Idiot!"

So you've got to break that habit. Better yet, break that belief system. If someone says you are attractive, you really don't have to try to talk them out of it. And if no one's telling you you're attractive, instead of automatically assuming it's because you're not hot enough, ask yourself what kind of "vibe" you're putting out there. If you reek of self-loathing, no one's going to want to come within ten feet of you—it's as simple as that. (And yes, we realize that "Stop hating yourself, already!" is not very practical, concrete advice, but that's what the rest of the book is for.)

WHAT'S YOUR TYPE?

Another thing to keep in mind is that very few people have types set in stone. Do we have preferences? Sure. But preferences are not hard-and-fast requirements. Marianne really likes tall guys, but her husband is under six feet. Her preference for tall was overridden by her preference for awesome. Likewise, her husband had never dated a fat woman before, but that didn't matter—because he also has a strong preference for awesomeness, and Marianne fit the bill. One of our friends got hitched last fall to an amazing guy she's absolutely gaga for—but for the first year they knew each other, she didn't feel a spark, because he wasn't her "type." It was just that the more she got to know him, the more her "type" shifted from whatever it was before to "someone exactly like him." Sometimes it works like that.

So we do suggest keeping an open mind. If someone who isn't your imaginary ideal shows an interest, ask yourself if you are automatically dismissing someone who could be a good partner just because they don't meet a standard you've dreamed up. Ignoring the guy at the end of the bar because he has a funny-looking nose isn't all that different from being dismissed by the guy at the other end of the bar because you're fat, you know?

Having said that, there are obviously some standards on which you don't want to compromise—and we would never recommend dating someone you don't feel any sexual chemistry with, just because he or she is there and willing. There are going to be people you're just not attracted to and never will be—and vice versa. These people do not make good long-term partners. But do evaluate if you are willing to compromise on *some* things. You know what else kept Kate single for ages? Her list of characteristics any potential partner would have to have: tall, funny, Ivy League–educated (even though she wasn't!), unflaggingly feminist, clean-shaven, bespectacled, nerdy-cute, gainfully employed in an artistic field (yeah, seriously), ready to live in either Canada or the States according to her dual-citizen whims, willing to consider being a stay-at-home dad . . . and it went on and on from there. That guy? Does not exist. Being willing to give a little will open up your dating pool a lot more than losing fifty pounds would.

PUTTING ONE FOOT IN FRONT OF THE OTHER

Of course, there's no guaranteed path to finding love, and if there were, it most likely wouldn't fit in a single chapter of a book. Believing that there are perfectly normal people who might be attracted to you, convincing yourself that you are worthy of love, behaving confidently, and relaxing your standards (a little!) will all go a long way toward attracting more potential partners. However, there are still factors you simply can't control.

There's the "S/he's just not that into you" factor—it does happen, and there ain't nothin' you can do about it, but move on.

There's the timing factor—Kate, for instance, has an uncanny gift for hitting it off with guys who are already partnered up.

But unless everyone involved is cheerfully polyamorous, *do not date people who aren't single.* It will shred your self-esteem, and then you'll just have to waste time reading this book all over again, when you could be meeting a new hottie (or your girlfriends) for cocktails.

And finally, there's the unfortunate reality of the culture we live in. Fact is, there might very well be people who do find you attractive but can't bring themselves to admit it. You know the website PostSecret.com, where people send in postcards revealing their deepest and darkest? (If you don't, you should. It's great.) One of the saddest secrets we've ever seen there was written in what we hope is the hand of a teenage boy who will grow up and develop the confidence never to do this to himself or a woman again: "I dumped you because my friends made fun of me for dating a FAT GIRL. But I am still in love with you." That is unbelievably shitty on so many levels, but you know what they say about shit: It happens. You're not the only one getting the cultural message that only sick freaks want to date fat women—we all are, fat and thin, men and women, gay and straight, and all shades in between those binaries. Resisting it takes a lot of strength and courage, whether you're the fat chick or the person who's attracted to one. And some people are just not up to the challenge. All you can do is make sure you are.

PART FOUR

{ AVOIDING NEGATIVITY }

CHAPTER THIRTEEN

Don't Hang Around with People Who
Say Negative Things About Your Body

Do you remember being a kid and coming home crying because someone said something mean to you on the playground? Maybe that particular childhood trauma didn't happen to everyone, but work with us here.

When you came home crying because someone said something mean to you, your caregiver of whatever flavor ought to have told you that people who say mean things to you are not your friends. It might have been a hard concept to grasp in kindergarten, because little Suzy had just shared her cookies with you the day before, and that meant you were best friends. But, playground politics being what they are, things changed, and you had to realize that and make some new friends.

Boy, do we wish everyone would remember this childhood lesson.

The friend who makes oinking noises when you go out to lunch together? Not your friend. The friend who insists you go clothes shopping with her as inspiration for you to lose weight? Not your friend. The friend who offers up commentary on how much larger your ass seems lately? Not your friend. And if those examples seem extreme, consider the friend who's always telling you about her diet—hint, hint. The friend who suggests you pick the dark-colored dress, because it's more slimming. The friend who looks askance at you if you order more than a small salad in a restaurant. Her behavior doesn't have to be so in-your-face to get the message across.

In adulthood, as in kindergarten, a person who is constantly engaged in tearing you down is not your friend. Friends build each other up. They support each other, and they want what is best for each other. "Do you really want to eat that?" is just the grown-up version of "You're an icky poopoo-head."

And, really, that is part of what can make navigating conversations about fat tricky—your so-called friend says she is concerned about your health, she just wants what is best for you, blah, blah, blah. But if that were true, she'd express it in a way that didn't shame you and attack your self-confidence. Once, after Kate had gained a bit of weight, she passed along a pair of kick-ass red capris to a friend of hers who was the right size for them. Instead of merely thanking her, the "friend" said, "Oh, don't worry, honey. We'll get you back into these!" Kate hadn't been worried—and, if she had been aiming to get back into those pants, there really wouldn't have been any "we" about it. But some women see their friends' weight as a group project, and they think they need to "help" a fatter friend by making subtle and not-so-subtle comments about her body. It's not helpful, and women like that are not good friends.

REAL CONCERNED FRIENDS

A lot of people also use a mask of concern for your health to put a more socially acceptable face on their fat hatred. But, remember, a real friend is not going to engage in behaviors that actively harm you. Genuine care and concern about your well-being is an awesome thing, and you should value a friend that comes to you in genuine concern and asks about your health. They want you to stick around! That's great! But there is a big difference between saying, "Hey, I'm concerned that your weight is having a negative impact on your health"—and then being prepared to listen and respect your answer, whatever it is—and "Hey, your big, fat ass is going to kill you one day!" (Marianne wishes she were making up that second example but, alas, some people's children just never learned any better.)

So, what do you do when faced with a friend who just can't seem to stop commenting on your food intake? First, we suggest standing up for yourself. You don't have to be rude, but you do have to be firm. Not saying anything won't change the situation, and it is possible that your friend doesn't realize what she or he is doing. Because, hey, we live in a diet- and body-obsessed culture where negative body talk is super common. It's possible he or she really doesn't realize how their commentary is making you feel.

How you have this conversation is up to you, of course. But we suggest not making a big deal about it, at least not at first. The next time your friend says, "You know, those pants really emphasize how stubby your legs are," try responding with, "You know, when you make comments like that, it's really painful to me. I'm happy with my body, and your negative commentary isn't helpful." This is a good time to apply non-confrontational language. It is not the time to bust out with, "You're a mean cow, and all that negative talking makes you sound like a horrible person."

If you have this conversation, and your friend puts some effort into no longer trashing your fat body, awesome! You've got a good friend there. But if your friend insists they aren't doing anything wrong and they are just trying to be helpful, and, you know, if you lost a little weight you wouldn't be so bitchy all the time . . . that person is not your friend.

If that's the case, as painful as it might be, you need to cut your ties with that person. Giving up a friend can be hard. It's like a breakup, and you will spend some time wondering if you've done the right thing or if you could salvage things and get back together. You might watch a lot of Sandra Bullock movies (Marianne's secret—well, not so secret anymore—remedy for truly sad times), and you might cry. All of that is okay.

Just try to remember, in the midst of it all, that you've done something to be proud of—you've taken care of your own mental health and put yourself first when it really counted. Because a "friend" who is willfully causing you emotional damage is no one who deserves to hang out with you. Another helpful thing to remember when you are feeling sad about the loss of your so-called friend is that there are lots of people out there that you haven't met yet who are going to think you are fantastic. You just have to get out there and meet them. This means talking to people in-person and online. It's where those hobbies that have nothing to do with your weight can really come in handy as well. Take the first step—invite that nice guy from pottery class to come hang out with you and your other friends at the bowling alley. Make a friendly date to go makeup shopping with the woman whose eye shadow is always perfect when you are volunteering together at the library.

ALL IN THE FAMILY

Of course, there are some people you can't get rid of. Although it is possible to cut ties entirely with family members, that isn't always a practical solution. And yet, family members, especially close family members, can push our buttons way more effectively than anyone else—after all, they installed those buttons to begin with! So what do you do?

Work on setting boundaries. If you've got an uncle who mentions your weight every single time you see him, it's time to let him know that you don't think that is acceptable. It's easy to convince ourselves not to stand up to family members, but setting boundaries means standing firm in your own defense.

It can also mean sitting down to have potentially awkward

conversations that no one really wants to have. When your mom mentions yet again how pretty you'd be if you just lost twenty pounds, you need to tell your mom that you are pretty exactly as you are and that you do not intend to discuss weight loss with her. Period. You don't have to flip out on her—again, nonconfrontational language usually works best in these situations—but you do have to be firm. "Mom, I appreciate your concern, but I am not willing to discuss my weight with you." And then change the subject.

Even if you don't appreciate her concern—because she's brought it up a thousand times—she probably thinks she is expressing how much she loves you by mentioning this stuff. We aren't sure how that logic works exactly, but that seems to be what mothers are getting at with comments like those. Keep that in mind when you respond. As much as she is driving you crazy, she loves you. It just doesn't mean she has a right to dictate what you do with your adult body.

Another thing you can change without even needing to have an uncomfortable conversation is the way you speak about your own body around family and friends. Making self-deprecating remarks about your fat thighs or your love handles sends people the message that you think such negative commentary is acceptable. Bitching about your back rolls gives other people permission to do it as well. And that's not cool.

None of this is easy. Dealing with family is especially straight-up difficult and scary. But by setting boundaries with family and friends, you are protecting your mental health. It is okay to take care of yourself. In fact, it is more than okay—it's necessary. Taking care of your needs is important and shouldn't be brushed aside out of the mistaken notion that others are more important than you are. Look at it this way: You wouldn't let someone say that crap to your best friend. Be your own best friend and don't let people say it to you either.

CHAPTER FOURTEEN

Don't Hang Around with People Who Say Negative Things About Their Own Bodies

Now that you aren't hanging out with people who say negative things about your body, you might start noticing that you know a lot of people who still say negative things about their own bodies. Sadly, this is just as uncool.

Other people will most likely have a problem if you bring up their own self-deprecating comments in discussion. After all, they'll argue, they aren't talking about *your* body! What does it matter what they say about their own bodies? Your body is fine.

Shame it never really seems to feel like that.

Marianne weighs more than a lot of her friends do (individually and, in some cases combined, ha!) and when those thinner friends complain about how fat they are, or how disgusting their bodies are, even though they don't intend it, there is an implied commentary being offered up on her own fatter body. After all, if someone who weighs a hundred pounds less thinks his or her body is wretched and appalling, how is it possible that Marianne's body is any better?

"I DON'T MEAN YOU!"

In our experience, the people who do this honestly believe that their self-loathing crap has no impact on other people. If you point out that your ass is twice as big as the one your friend is disparaging, she'll say something like, "Oh, but you always look great! I don't mean you! I just don't like how I look!" Well, that's swell, but you just said you're too fat, and I am obviously way fatter. On what freakin' planet is that not a comment on my body, too?

Friends who do this may be suffering from serious body dysmorphia, or they may just have their heads stuck up their not-so-fat asses. Either way, it's toxic. You can't police how your friends feel about themselves, nor should you be able to. But, once again, you can choose with whom you spend your time.

Now, some of you, dear readers, might be thinking we intend for you to ditch everyone you know and either spend all your time alone with the cats or start from scratch acquiring friends and acquaintances. Truly, though, we're not suggesting you cut off everyone you love. We just want you to know that you deserve friends and acquaintances who aren't going to make you feel like shit—and that those people really do exist.

CONTAGIOUS

The big problem with hanging out with people who are constantly offering up negative monologues about their own bodies is that it's contagious. It's nearly impossible to hang around someone who's always harping on her body flaws, real or perceived, and not start critiquing your own body. If you are surrounding yourself with negativity, well, even though this sounds a little New Agey, know it is that much easier to fall into negativity yourself.

Imagine it, you're out with your friend, and she says, "God, I hate my arms so much. I could never wear a sleeveless shirt." Now, you don't see anything wrong with her arms, but you start to wonder about your own. Or you are already having a little trouble feeling comfortable when you bare your arms and, well, if her arms aren't good enough to go sleeveless, there's no way you're going to try on that tank top. Pass the long-sleeved T-shirt, please.

So now you're stuck having to have another awkward conversation. We're asking a lot, we know, but we promise it will help. Next time you and your friend are on that shopping trip and she starts talking about her body, gently point out that her negative commentary really brings you down. You don't have to make a big deal of it, but you should begin to point out, each time it happens, how negative your friend is being about her body. And if she can't change, you might need to find a new shopping partner.

This is a situation in which setting a good example, as cheesy as it sounds, can really help. If you aren't talking trash about your body, if you are praising yourself and focusing on how awesome you are, that might just rub off on your friend.

If it doesn't, it isn't a personal failure. Your positive messages can only do so much to counteract all the negative messages we are being fed by the media. Unless your friends jump on the self-acceptance bandwagon along with you, there is a limited amount that you can do. You can't force them to love their bodies; but maybe you can at least get them to shut up about hating their pudgy elbows.

CHAPTER FIFTEEN

Don't Participate in Diet Talk

"They," in all their infinite wisdom, say that nothing brings people together like a crisis. Maybe this is why so many women bond over diet talk. The deprivation and mental toll that come from not eating enough certainly count as a crisis situation for your body!

We've noticed that if you put a group of average women together at a restaurant, the talk will most likely turn to how many calories the women have consumed or burned, how many pounds they "need" to lose, what size they were when they were eighteen years old, and what size they think they're going to be when they're through with the latest in a long series of diets. Instead of savoring the food they are paying for, these women talk about how "bad" or how "good" they are being, how hard it is to resist the real butter for their bread, or the bread itself, blah, blah, blah.

And then the dessert tray comes out and the real self-recrimination begins!

Y'all, this is fucked up. Such behavior is so ridiculous and full of self-loathing that we can hardly believe people voluntarily engage in it—much less consider an evening spent this way a good time.

Too many women substitute diet talk for real conversation. They use it to bond, but it is a superficial bond that undermines the chance of any real connection. It pretends to align women as sisters working toward a common goal, but it really turns them into competitors. Who lost the most this week? Who gained weight? Who ordered salad dressing on the side? Who's going to do an extra hour at the gym tomorrow to justify ordering an appetizer? Who just can't seem to resist the amazing molten chocolate cake?

Don't be one of those women, okay? When faced with a decadent dessert, remember what we've said about intuitive eating, and decide if you want it based on what your body tells you. (Are you still hungry? Are you craving something sweet? Do you just want to taste it, but not eat a lot—in which case, you are allowed to throw most of it away, even if you can't dragoon a friend into sharing? Do you feel like you could, quite happily, eat the whole thing and feel neither overfull nor overdosed on sugar? All of those possibilities are fine—you just need to check in with your body, instead of the part of your brain that determines whether eating dessert would be a social liability.) And when faced with a menu, don't order a salad because it seems like the virtuous, low-calorie choice. Choose it because you have been craving the crisp earthiness of baby field greens or the crunch of garlic herb croutons. And if you're not craving those things, don't order the freakin' salad.

Choose what you want to eat and choose something else to talk about. You're going to blaze new trails here. You're going to lead these women (and some men as well) into the exciting waters of actual conversation!

AT THE RESTAURANT

The next time you're out to dinner and someone mentions that there is just no way she could possibly eat that, you have a choice. You can let the comment itself slide and change the subject, or you can challenge the person by asking her why she can't allow herself to have something she so clearly wants.

If you take the first tack, you are probably going to have to change the subject several times during the meal. This meal, and the next meal, and probably the next meal, too. That's okay if you have patience and this sort of nonconfrontational thing is more your speed. Come to eat prepared with interesting stories, questions you can ask your dinner companions, and a lot of patience for the inevitable "bad" food comments that will be made. Kate recently had dinner with two old friends, who knew full well that she writes a body acceptance blog and was working on this book, and she still had to navigate around conversations about the evils of white rice, how young people today won't even take the stairs instead of the elevator, and how an hour at the gym every day just didn't seem to be enough to make one thin friend lose weight. Kate wasn't in the mood to get on her soapbox that night, so she just kept shutting her mouth and changing the subject as necessary.

If you are fed up with being subtle, though—and you are willing to risk not being invited out to dinner with these people again—it's time to be a bit more direct. The next time someone says, "Oh, I am being good, I'm on a diet," ask them "Why do you attach moral virtue to your food? Do you believe that eating mashed potatoes would really make you a bad person?" Talk about awkward conversations. Especially if this is one of those "friends" who is always commenting on what you eat. Marianne had dinner once with new friends. She had never met Stephanie before, and when the waiter took drink orders, Stephanie ordered water. Marianne, making conversation, asked if she didn't drink. Stephanie replied with a laugh, "No, I'm pregnant. I'm not always this fat." Marianne laughed and said in reply, "Oh, I'm always this fat. I'm just fat." Awkward! But funny in retrospect and, in subsequent dinners, Stephanie has never used "fat" in a negative way.

You probably have more tact than Marianne. But even if you don't, nixing diet talk at the table really does make for a more pleasant dining experience.

MYSPACE AND OTHER SPACES

Unfortunately, diet talk isn't limited to dinner out with your girlfriends. It happens in the office, in online communities, and in the mall over fitting room walls. Although you can't completely insulate yourself from it, you can work to eradicate it from your own spaces. If you have a blog, like Kate and Marianne, let your readers know that it's an anti-diet talk space.

If your online friends are talking about their diets, skip those entries and explain why you won't be reading them. Tell the women at the office that you're sorry, you don't believe in dieting, so you can't join them for lunch unless they will be talking about something else. Refuse to join company-wide competitions to see who can lose the most weight, and—if you think you can do so without jeopardizing your position—let the higher-ups know that these kinds of "wellness" programs can be terribly damaging to people with a history of disordered eating, to say nothing of garden variety fat people.

This one takes guts, no doubt about it. But the more you let people know that you aren't going to tolerate their constant chattering about self-deprivation, the less they'll turn to you for that conversation. Chances are good that it will feel refreshing for them, too.

CHAPTER SIXTEEN

Seek Out Images of Happy, Healthy, Hot, Fat Women

You turn on the TV, and every woman you see is a size 0. You open a magazine, and ditto. You go to the mall, and you see new clothes displayed on tiny mannequins in the windows of stores that don't even carry your size. If all you see when you look at the world is women who are thin, it's really easy to start feeling like your body is just too big for this world.

Given what is by now an old saw, that the average American woman wears a size 14 (meaning 50 percent of us wear a bigger size than that), it's absurd to look at very thin women as the norm, and everyone else as an outlier. But we do. The problem is, it's really easy to go through an entire day where you only interact with a few actual women, yet see dozens of *images* of women, all of whom are thin. And that can start to make you feel like you and your fat ass just don't belong. Of course *all* of us belong, no matter what our size, but it can be hard to remember that when our cultural image of a "normal" weight is actually much smaller than what's most common or even healthiest. (Fun fact: The "overweight" BMI category is actually the one with the lowest mortality rates of all—lower than "normal."[1]) Very thin people are neither typical of the population nor necessarily any healthier than the rest of us. Just like very fat people, they've got a body type that's at the edge of the bell curve, while most folks fall somewhere in the middle. The media just makes it seem as though that rare body type is quite common.

PAINTED LADIES (AND OTHER PEOPLE, TOO)

There are so many different kinds of bodies out there. And, though you'd never know it from looking at fashion spreads, there are lots of different skin tones, too. Now you just need the visuals to prove it. If you are a fat person (or a person of color or a person who is differently abled or a person who just doesn't jibe with the current popular style) you are going to need to turn to alternate sources for your images of normality.

Of course there is nothing wrong with models and actresses. But if you're not tall and willowy, they aren't representative of you. They aren't representative of your neighbor down the street, either (well, maybe if you live in L.A.). Just keep in mind—what we see the most is what we consider the norm. Branching out to include women of other shapes and sizes will remind you that you're a normal human being, not a hippopotamus.

Where can you find these alternate sources? All over the

place! First, go to the park and watch the women who walk by. They will have all sorts of bodies and skin tones and ability levels. Remind yourself that all of these women are perfectly normal—and the women who represent the cultural beauty ideal are rare. (Which is not to say weird or freakish or any of the other epithets applied to the very fat and very thin alike. Just statistically outside the norm.)

One of the most powerful things you can do to fight the homogenous image of Woman being presented by the mainstream media is to stop consuming that mainstream media. We don't mean you can never go to another movie, but we highly recommend that you stop reading some of the most popular women's magazines, unless you're really bored at the salon. You know the ones we're talking about. The ones that tell you to love yourself but then give you three more articles explaining how to camouflage that "unfortunate" tummy bulge. Put those down and don't pick them back up. Following the latest fashion trends is not worth inflicting this crap on yourself. And if you just can't live without a magazine to take with you to the doctor's waiting room, check out magazines like Bust and Bitch, which, while they aren't explicitly fat-positive, do try to tackle the world from a feminist perspective. Your psyche will thank you.

Then it's time to branch out. If you like classical Art with a capital A, there are a number of painters who preferred to paint and sculpt large bodies. You no doubt know the term Rubenesque was derived from Peter Paul Rubens's later paintings—but have you checked out those paintings? His voluptuous figures are exuberantly baroque and were inspired by his young wife, Helene. Or, if baroque nudes are not to your taste, check out the paintings and sculptures by Fernando Botero. This Colombian artist is famous for his portraits of fat people—much to the chagrin of some critics. His sculptures are large in all ways, towering over people with their generous flesh. Botero has also been quite vocal about what he's doing—he's trying to create beauty. There is no ambiguity in his intentions when it comes to his fat people.

If you like your art a little more photographic, you are in even more luck. Did you know that Leonard Nimoy, Mr. Spock from the original *Star Trek* series (not to be confused with Dr. Spock, famous pediatrician), is also a photographer who has focused on fat bodies with his Full Body Project? Another of our favorite artists is Laurie Toby Edison. Her Women en Large project is nothing short of life changing for many viewers. And for a little bit of sexy in your photographs, check out Substantia Jones's Adipositivity Project—which is definitely not safe for work, but can inspire you to look at your body in a new light. (We should note that the Adipositivity Project has received some fair criticism for not highlighting very many women of color, but Substantia was taking some steps to diversify the project as we were writing this.)

Why haven't you heard of these artists before? Probably because the media is busy focusing on women who have a body type that only about 2 percent of the population can come by naturally. That's the body that diet industry wants you to consider normal. After all, that's how they make their money.

FAT PEOPLE ARE EVERYWHERE—
AND SO ARE FAT-POSITIVE IMAGES

The fact that you are not a freak becomes a lot more evident the more you surround yourself with non-mainstream representations of women. And these representations don't have to come from art. Get out into your community. Join fat-positive communities online. We don't just mean our blogs! Whether you are browsing Livejournal or flipping through back issues of *Mode* (our favorite plus size mag ever, now sadly defunct) or new issues of *Skorch*, there are awesome images of fat people everywhere. Check out the Fatshionista blog and community on Livejournal. You'll see pictures of fabulous fatties every single day with all sorts of different fashion styles. Visit online plus-size retailers' sites, even if you can't afford the clothes— shops like Igigi, B and Lu, and Junonia often feature women of much larger sizes than even the typical plus-size model. Do a tag search on Flickr.com for three hundred pounds and check out what pops up (hint: A lot of these photos are Lesley, of Fatshionista.com). Fans of sculpture might want to sift through Stephanie Metz's portfolio. Her wool felt bodies (of different sizes) are pretty amazing.

Unfortunately, we can't provide an extensive and detailed list of resources across every artistic medium. The truth is that sometimes it can be hard to find fat people involved in contemporary, mainstream artistic endeavors. Art reflects culture, and our culture is, well, you know what it is. Keep your eyes open, and you'll find stuff, but the resources change a lot. Start with what we've listed and treat it like an adventure or a scavenger hunt. And then let us know what you find!

When you seek out images of awesome, happy, active fat people, you start to realize there are a lot more of us than TV, movies, and magazines would suggest. And that really can inspire you to believe that you can be one, too. Who knows—you might even wind up contributing to the Fatshionista Flickr pool and inspiring someone else.

PART FIVE

{ Getting Dressed }

CHAPTER SEVENTEEN

Make Friends with a Tailor/Learn to Sew

You find an amazingly cute and perfect dress—it's on sale, to boot!—and you take it to the fitting room with the highest of hopes, only to have those hopes dashed against the floor because this dress, the dress of your dreams, doesn't fit right. It clings in the stomach, and the straps are too long, and the boobs are too small or too big, and it hits at the wrong length, and—who designs these clothes, anyway?

In such situations it is easy to get angry with your body. If only it were the right shape, you think, clothes would fit properly. If only your breasts were the right size, your legs were longer, your arms thinner. If only.

But your body is a living thing, and clothes are inanimate objects. Your body changes while that pair of pants stays the same. And your body is different from the body of the woman in the next stall over. She's having trouble with that dress, too, but probably not the same trouble you're having.

It seems elementary but it is important to be reminded sometimes: Every body is different. Your body is not the problem. The clothes are the problem.

READY TO WEAR VERSUS BESPOKE

A little bit of fashion industry history: The concept of ready-to-wear is actually fairly recent in the scope of humans wearing clothes. The rise of the department store didn't hit until the mid-to late 1920s and even after that, during the Depression, it was common for people to make their own garments. The very wealthy have always had clothes custom-made for a reason—custom-made clothes fit better and look better. And custom-made clothes also wear better and last longer, because they don't suffer the stresses that clothes that "sort of" fit do. Unfortunately, people stopped passing on sewing knowledge as a life skill. And custom-made clothes are expensive. Ready-to-wear filled that gap with stylish pieces that were available much more cheaply and with a lot more instant gratification.

Of course, the difficulty of ready-to-wear is that it has to be designed to fit an average body type and to be wearable by a lot of different bodies that all sort of conform to the same size and shape. Thus the fit model, as the term is currently used, came into existence, much to the frustration of women everywhere.

A fit model is a woman—usually several are employed by any given designer or brand of women's clothing—who serves as the average figure for which clothes are designed. Because there is no standardization in women's clothing sizes, fit models are the sole guides for many designers. A designer's line is then scaled up or down, often by computer, from the fit model's measurements to draft patterns for other sizes. Even plus-size clothing manufacturers usually build their lines around "a perfect size 18"—so if you're any other size, or an imperfect 18, they won't always be quite right on you.

What this means is that, quite literally, clothes are not designed to fit your body. So say it with us once more: Your body is not the problem—the clothes are.

Even if you've found a brand that usually fits, you're not necessarily home free. Clothing designs are sent to factories all over the world for manufacturing. Two different colors of the same pair of pants may not fit the same because they were sent to two different factories with two different margins of error. The two garments may only differ by a quarter of an inch, but in clothing, that quarter of an inch can have a big impact.

There is hope. Because designers all use different fit models, you might find one brand that fits as though it really were made for you. And if you can find something close, even better—alterations can perfect the fit of your new garment.

VIEW A OR VIEW B?

So, what are your options (other than looking like a hot mess)? Well, that strap that keeps falling down is a five-minute sewing job or a couple of dollars to a tailor. That dress that is too big? Taking it in will improve the look of it and extend the garment's life. For some reason, a lot of women are resistant to the idea of alterations, although in higher-end stores, including department stores, this service is both expected and often used. A lot of people are put off by the imagined cost of alterations, but keep in mind that some stores offer them for free, and your dry cleaner can probably do simple jobs for a few dollars. If you factor in prolonged life of the garment and better fit, the extra cost may well be worthwhile anyway.

Some alterations can be done at home quickly and easily, even if you've never picked up a sewing needle before. Do you have a button up shirt that fits like a dream except for the spot where it gaps between the second and third buttons? Find a needle and thread that matches your garment, sit down in a well-lighted area, and use small stitches to sew that area up. It means you'll have to pull the button-up over your head, but you'll have another shirt that you can wear without embarrassment. An alternative to sewing is to use a very small safety pin to catch a few bits of the fabric so that you can pin the gap closed. (This is a far more temporary solution and you'll need to take the safety pins out before laundering the shirt to avoid rust.)

Do you have a strap on a dress that keeps falling down? Try the dress on, measure how much slack you need to take up in the straps and either pin the straps at the new length or permanently sew them down by hand.

Pants that gap at the back waist? This fix is a little more complex and involves taking a few darts. Unless you are already comfortable with a needle and thread, you'll want to take this to a seamstress. Ask a local dry cleaner for recommendations if you don't know who to trust. Dry cleaners work with seamstresses and tailors on a frequent basis, and they know good work when they see it.

Of course, as Marianne likes to point out, you can also learn to make your own clothes. You don't need super expensive and fancy tools to craft custom garments that suit both your body and your style. All you need is a basic sewing machine—and a source of sewing knowledge. This can be classes (often taught in sewing shops and big-box craft stores), books, or a friend or family member who can sew. Although sewing is not always as economical as bargain shopping (some fabrics and trims are crazy expensive), the custom fit makes it worth the effort.

And when sewing from patterns—which is not a requirement if you understand basic garment construction—be aware that you might have to make adjustments for garments to fit you. Sewing is a very individual process, which can sometimes be frustrating. The rewards, though, are a fantastic wardrobe that no one else has.

The reward is also a wardrobe that fits *you* and fits you *well.* Clothes that fit you well do not have to be figure-conscious or tight in any way, but they do have to be the right size. Garments, even store-bought items, are designed with a certain amount of "ease." Ease is the difference between the garment measurements and your measurements. If you are wearing clothes with too much ease, your clothes are too big—you might feel like the extra room is hiding your fat, but usually, it just makes you look sloppy. If you don't know your size, take a good, honest, nonjudgmental friend with you to the mall and try on clothes across a span of sizes. Clothes that are too tight will be uncomfortable, and clothes that are too big will gap and bunch in funny ways or otherwise look like a tent. (If you're trying on trapeze dresses, of course, it's possible to totally rock that tent look. Our friend Lesley, of Fatshionista.com, is a staunch defender of the trapeze dress, and she makes a good point that's relevant to a lot of women whose bodies don't match the cultural ideal: "These are garments that are, unbelieveably, cut to fit my *actual* shape. Cue the laughter when I so often see people exclaim that only the impossibly slender—that is, those whose shape is the categorical opposite of the trapeze dress itself—can successfully wear them.")

Whether you find that perfectly fitted garment from just the right designer, by visiting a tailor, or by learning to sew, your clothes will suit you much better when they fit your actual body. Remember, it isn't your fault when clothes don't fit. Our cardinal rule of shopping: *Don't blame yourself—blame the garment!* Toss that little dress back to the fitting room attendant and find something that rocks on the body you've got.

"I can't drive in this Jacket!"
And Other Reasons to Blame the Fit Model

by Joy Nash

So one day, about three years ago, I stumbled across a fit model measurement chart on the Internet and much to my surprise, realized that I was an "exact size 18." I googled "Fit Model Agency," walked in a week later, and got signed. For reals, it was that easy. Once I was signed, my agency had me take a crash course in fit modeling so I wasn't completely clueless and then started sending me out on interviews.

For the unititiated: A fit model provides a kind of baseline frame of reference for a designer to work from. If you're not a fit model (or don't have the exact same measurements as one), then clothing off the rack is not going to fit you perfectly. Sucks, but there's really no other economical choice. Those of us who are fit models are basically live mannequins for pattern-makers and designers. We're "proportionate"—which means more hour-glassy than super-booby or pear-shaped—and generally 5'5" to 5'8" (any taller and you'll need a "tall" size, any shorter and you'll be "petite.") We're also usually a size 18, or 2X, because that's close to the middle of the range of sizes that the clothes are going to hit the stores in: 14/16, 18/20, 22/24, 26/28 or 0X, 1X, 2X, 3X, 4X.

Once the pattern is approved in an 18, it'll be graded up and down through the rest of the sizes. A fit model is responsible for trying on samples and bringing any fit issues to the designer's attention. We say things like: "I can't lift my arms. I think the shoulder seam should be let out," or "These jeans need a longer zipper. I can't even get them over my hips like this." Basically, we're paid (quite well) to stay the exact same size and let the designers in on the 3-D aspects of the garment—things they can't see in a 2-D sketch or rendering.

Once the designer has made her notes and the fit model has made her suggestions, adjustments are made, a new sample is sewn up, and the model is brought in for another fitting. And on it goes, sometimes through three or four revisions before a sample is approved and sent into production.

Within both plus and straight categories there are junior and missy (or contemporary) sizing. A junior plus fit model is usually a 1X, or size 16, and measures bust: 40.5–41.5, waist: 33–34, hips: 43–44. Junior plus is the stuff you'll find at Torrid, Fashion Bug, and lots of those cheap strip mall stores that carry "Big Size." Junior plus sizing figures you have slightly smaller boobs, prefer a lower rise on your jeans, and generally want things to be brighter, louder, and more closely fitted. Also, junior sizing is often in odd numbers: 13, 15, 17; whereas missy is always on the evens: 14, 16, 18.

Missy sizing is a little more generous. It expects you to have larger boobs, a semi-defined waist, and a hip measurement about ten inches larger than your waist measurment. A missy size 18 typically measures bust: 45–49, waist: 36–41.5, hips: 47–51. Missy is the sizing you'll find at department stores like Nordstrom and Macy's and in the more mature styles at Lane Bryant and the Avenue. Also, anything with a *W* behind the number: (14W, 24W) is definitely in missy size.

Total product plug, but one of my very first fit clients was Paige Premium Denim—and honestly I struck gold when they chose me.

Paige Premium is designed by Paige Adams-Gellar, who worked for years as a fit model herself for denim labels like True Religion, Seven for All Mankind, Guess, and Lucky Brand—all famous for a fabulous fit—before starting her own line. And naturally, Paige Premium Denim is now famous in the straight size world for having an incredible fit. Like Kate says, I've got horseshoes up my ass (making me the luckiest girl in the world), so Paige picked me to be the fit model when she expanded her line into plus sizes.

I remember the first few fittings I had, I'd try on the jeans and think they looked pretty friggin' great. But the woman makes the big bucks because she's a perfectionist. She'd look at me and say the pockets need to be at a quarter of an inch tilt; the thighs let out a quarter; the hips, three-eighths of an inch smaller. I'd stand there thinking, "But wait! What about the girl whose hips are three-eighths of an inch bigger than mine! She'll love these jeans!" But, as I came to learn, that's not the point. If the jeans are made fit to the curvier girl, then the more straight-up-and-down girl will have seas of fabric to deal with. If we're fitting to the flat butt, booty city isn't gonna be able to get the damn things up her legs. They were making the jeans to fit me, and I needed to give the feedback that would allow them to create a pair of pants perfectly tailored to my body. This (unfortunately) was not the moment to advocate for the masses.

Fitting is about finding a happy medium. Because it's not feasible to fit every garment to fifteen different girls and average the differences between them all, the designer just has to pick one body that is close to the median and fit to her. So until everybody is designing like Lane Bryant's Right Fit line, with different fits for different body shapes, you gotta get thee to a sewing machine!

CHAPTER EIGHTEEN

Buy Fabulous Clothes and Wear Them

This ought to be the shortest chapter in the book. Because, really, what you need to know—and firmly believe—is that there is practically no excuse for buying clothes you don't love. If your clothing budget is tight, or you wear a size that limits your options even within the plus market, finding clothes you love can certainly be a lot harder than it is for other people. But it's still not impossible.

We've observed that too many fat women—even those who aren't limited much by size or budget—will buy *anything* that fits. Even if they don't like it. Even if it isn't what they were looking for in the first place. There is such a relative scarcity of clothing for fat women that finding something in your size, something merely "good enough," can feel like a major shopping triumph. But we do not believe in settling for "good enough." We believe in seeking out great. If you purchase something that you don't love, you are shorting yourself. You deserve clothes that make you feel awesome.

So, that satin skirt with the mermaid cut that you found on clearance and passed up anyway because you "won't ever have anywhere to wear it"? That wicked power suit that's a little much for your current job? Buy them! Buy (or make!) clothes that make you excited to be getting dressed—that attitude will shine through and make you look even more fabulous than the clothes.

And that old axiom about it being better to have a few expensive pieces than a hundred cheap ones? If you really, really love those few expensive pieces, then it is absolutely true.

This isn't true just because we say it is. It's true because of the concept of cost-per-wear. What does that mean? It means that, for instance, you find a dress you adore for $100, and you buy it. Then you wear it once a week for the next year. Meanwhile, you find another dress that costs $20. You buy it, but you only wear it twice in the next year. That hundred dollar dress breaks down to just under two bucks you have invested per wear. Meanwhile, the dress that seemed like such a bargain at $20? Each wear cost you $10, because you just didn't love it enough to wear it.

Suddenly, that hundred dollar dress seems like a much better deal.

The goal, remember, is to start living now. Not when (if) you are ever a size 6. Living now means not punishing yourself with an empty or otherwise lacking closet. Buy and wear clothes that make you feel terrific—and it doesn't matter if that means super femme dresses every day of the week or a collection of dark wash jeans that suit you and your needs to a tee.

Of course, we love shopping, and we know that not everyone does. If you hate it, today's your lucky day, because you get to benefit from the knowledge of the plus-size clothing market we've gained after years of trial and error—check out the appendix on plus-size retailers in the back of the book. Especially if you're willing to shop online, there are a lot more options out there, for every budget, than most women realize. For store reviews, you might also want to visit Fatshionista .com, where a constantly updated comprehensive list of retailers is maintained, along with actual customer experiences and ratings.

Now get out there and wear what you love!

Thrift Tips for Fatties

by Cynara Geissler

The shop reviews on fat-o-sphere sites like Fatshionista.com and the Fatshionista community on LiveJournal.com are amazing resources for locating the latest fatshions online and in brick and mortar stores. Certainly the pleasure of slipping into a crisp, brand-spanking-new-with-tags garment cannot be denied, but neither can the special satisfaction of discovering a lovely one-of-a-kind dress among racks of Cosby sweaters and faded Mickey Mouse T-shirts.

In general, when I covet a certain piece, I will take to secondhand and thrift stores first. I believe that as a society we (myself firmly included) produce too much, consume too much, and waste even more. So, I thrift (when possible), not only because I have a deep and abiding love for indestructible polyester and vintage pieces, but because I can more easily justify a sizable wardrobe if a large portion of it is made up of more recycled clothing. Thrifting is one of the ways I can personally contribute (if in a microscopic way) to a healthier planet (and prevent myself from literally having to live in my shoes). By now some of you are saying, "Hey, Cynara, I kind of agree with you, and I'd really love to get more into thrifting but . . . given the scarcity of fun and fatshionable things that I'd actually want to wear in stores that are supposed to stock my size, how can I reasonably expect not to be utterly demoralized and disappointed in a venue that isn't explicitly fattie-friendly?"

I won't deny that shopping and scarcity is a persistent issue in the fat-o-sphere. I can't guarantee that thrifting will never be difficult and discouraging and demoralizing when you're outside what the fashion industry/majority of retailers dub the "normal" size range. I will also freely admit that I'm fortunate because in my city (and neighborhood) there are quite a few thrift stores, and the majority of them even have plus-size sections. What's more, the flexibility of my current job and my general love of the chase make thrifting viable for me. Some days I have amazing luck. Other days, it feels like the loveliest pieces never exist in double digits, and I end up trolling disposable mall stores and department store sales for pieces that elude me in the secondhand shops and will fit and still allow me to pay my rent. I don't have a solution for thrifting woes, but, for me, the rewards of thrifting trump the frustrations and are not just limited to the sartorial. To encourage those of you who've got one foot on the thrifted (and fabulous!) wagon to climb aboard and go the distance, I've assembled some thrift tips.

Thrift Tip the First: Try Shit On

This might seem really, *really* obvious, but one of the tragic flaws of shoppers of all sizes (like Shakespearean characters) is that we don't look at the actual physical dimensions of a garment but believe that its "fitliness" corresponds directly to the number on the tag. If a lovely catches our eye, we immediately find the tag, and if the number on it proves to be smaller or—god forbid!—*larger* than the (arbitrary and usually inconsistent) number we think we wear, we—more often than not—dejectedly let it sink back into the secondhand depths. I am, according to most plus-size retailers, in the 18/20/22 range, but I've got things in my closet ranging from size 10 to 26 that *fit*. I would never have discovered half of these things if I confined my search to the (singular and usually hideously fugly) rack labeled "Plus."

Thrift stores are great places to build up your shopping courage/ fattitude. I have never once had anyone in a thrift store stop me from trying something on, and I think that's where what friends refer to as "my bizarre sense of shopping entitlement" comes from. You can treat thrift stores like giant fitting rooms and (in my experience) no one will bat an eye. There are few among us who haven't experienced a derisive remark from a salesclerk or had other shoppers take shots at us for our size. I think the fear and memory and expectation of this sort of behavior—the huge amount of ill-fitting crap notwithstanding— makes shopping stressful and emotionally trying. Being able to pull and grab stuff off racks and try them on on the spot in thrift shops has proved gratifying and liberating for me. It has greatly improved my eye for what will fit my body and it also reaffirms just how wildly sizes vary, which has helped me not to be attached to a number and attach meaning—negative or positive—to that number, but rather to focus on *what fits*.

Thrift Tip the Second: Find a Fat Thrift Buddy/ Form a Dynamic Duo

I begin this tip with an astute observation from Fatshionista.com's Lesley: "I think a lot of nonactivist fat-friendships are based on collaboratively dieting and/or 'supporting' one another in the apparent misery of fatness—I think taking a fat friend and forming a positive Dynamic Duo to conquer the Fat Thrift Challenge is wonderfully inspirational in a non-body-hating way."

And how.

Many of us have had friendships where we enabled body-hatred and negativity, and nowhere is this hatred more actively played out than during clothes shopping. Your mileage may vary, but many of my mall-trolling days were spent with girls much smaller than I, though we all hated and resented our bodies with equal intensity. When things fit, we still found a way to put a negative spin on it: "This is cute but would be better if I had more/less [insert body part here] . . ." I don't think a day went by when we didn't talk about how much weight we felt we should lose. Even if you somehow escaped those let's-bond-over-insulting-our-bodies conversations, you've no doubt overheard them in fitting rooms, clothing stores, and public washrooms.

The context in which these relationships are established—one of a shared body hate and shame—is far from empowering.

Finding a fat friend to thrift with is, on the other hand, a really fantastic premise to build on and revolutionary for a lot of us. Just imagine how much more navigable clothes hunting is when you're going at it with someone you can bitch with about the lack of options (rather than lamenting your body proper) and celebrate with when you find something incredible. (Another fattie will *totally* get the exhilaration of finding a mint-condition fifties housedress in your size and will probably squee right along with you.)

And let's not ignore the tactical and time-saving advantages of a shopping companion! Your friend can hit up cardigans, while you scour dresses; you can scope out skirts, while they plow through pants. If you're close in size, you can search for two. If you're different sizes, it's not a big deal. The friend doesn't have to be fat—they just have to be an actual friend (that is, not negative or mocking your body or size).

I have a fat friend who I thrift with on a regular basis, and I wouldn't have it any other way. Our styles and sizes aren't exactly the same, but we know each other's tastes and body types so well that we can grab stuff for each other. There are a few thrift stores in my area that border on warehouse size, and I couldn't imagine tackling them solo. And I know I don't need to tell you that trying on a velvet sequined jumpsuit with gigantic shoulder pads when you're by yourself is vaguely amusing when recounted—trying it on in front of your friend (who may or may not have a camera phone) becomes a legend for the ages!

Thrifting with a fellow fatty doesn't mean every day will be a good body day. But, if you're blessed with (fat) friends like mine, you'll find they are awesome at acknowledging that loving and appreciating your body in this fat-hating culture can be tough, while refusing to let you perpetrate active self-hate.

Thrift Tip the Third: Don't Be Afraid to Negotiate the Price

Props to Fatshionista.com reader Olivia Mae, whose email helped me flesh out this tip. She writes: "I work at a thrift shop . . . [and] wanted to pass on some tips . . . if you spot something with a small hole/stain or a bit of wear and tear, simply point it out to me, and I might possibly give you a small discount."

In my years of thrifting, I've found that prices do tend to be steep, given the quality/wear and tear of many of the items. In fact, high cost, besides the incredible scarcity of plus-size items, is probably the most common complaint voiced to me whenever I open dialogues about thrifting. Used clothing has become so pricey, people tell me, that one is better off shopping clearance at box stores, because there you'll get *new* clothing for the price of what you'd pay for something pre-loved—and you're guaranteed selection.

The way I address wear and tear (the only way you can, in my honest opinion) is pretty straightforward: I *politely* point out garment flaws and stains to a salesperson, and they, more often than not, adjust the total to something more reasonable. Call me callous, but given the coldhearted capitalist culture we live in, I tend to take the position that most stores and companies are (if inadvertently) prepared to soak me for as much as possible, and, I dare say, *rip me off*. Thus, I'm of the mind that when it comes to shopping for clothing, it behooves me to shift things more to my liking, both in terms of price and employee/customer interactions.

I won't say that thrifting is all *Let's Make a Deal* all the time, because I don't believe the prices are *always* unfair. But if you've spent any amount of time in a large thrift department store (especially chains like Value Village or Savers), you've probably noticed that pricing from store to store (and even week to week) can be wildly inconsistent. At giant stores, the volume of donations is large, and they try to price and replenish racks quickly. They do the best they can in the time they have, but anyone who's worked in retail knows how fast things move. Pricers and sorters don't always have time to comb garments for imperfections and are generally pricing based on like items and brand reputation. It seems reasonable to assume that in these circumstances some items will end up priced high. (The opposite is also true . . . every now and then designer labels are priced ridiculously low. These rare finds constitute the Thrifting Holy Grail, but that's a tip for another time).

If you operate under the philosophy that humans are fallible, bargaining isn't necessarily about being stingy—it's a way to actively engage in the often unthinking and automatic act of purchase exchange (I know I often "check out" at the check out, absently punching in the PIN on my debit card before even looking at the total . . . very unsettling) and keep thrift prices reasonable and competitive.

This tip might get some backs up, because many thrift shops and secondhand stores are run by charities (the Salvation Army, for instance) or donate a portion of their proceeds to charity. Although

I'm not exactly flush with cash, I don't mind paying more for second-hand items (after all, fine vintage pieces fetch scads on eBay), when I know my consumer indulgence will go to a good cause.

Olivia Mae closed her email reminding us that being nice to store employees is beneficial not just for obtaining an occasional discount, but also for tracking down coveted items. She notes, "I can easily help you find things, since I probably put the clothes on the racks . . . [and] if we don't have a particular something that you had in mind, then I might just keep my eye out for you in the sorting room when I am tagging and pricing clothes."

I know I often frame thrifting as a sort of a wo/man versus environment conflict. Racks upon (often disorganized) racks of potential allies and enemies that I (and my fat thrift friend) must conquer on my (our) own. I forget that staff are there to help and could point me in the right direction when I'm after something specific! Thank you, Olivia, for that reminder.

CHAPTER NINETEEN

Don't Shop at Stores That Don't Carry Your Size (Even If You Are with Thin Friends)—and Tell Them You're Not Shopping There

We've all been there. And by there, we mean at the mall with thinner friends, wandering around stores that don't stock our size, reduced to looking at earrings, while our friends try on stacks of clothes.

Now, maybe you're at the mall with those friends, and it seems like the thing to do, hanging out while they try on clothes. But—and this might be a little controversial—it is more important to take care of your mental health than it is to reassure your friend that, yes, that miniskirt looks fantastic on her. It's possible that going into stores that only carry straight sizes doesn't bother you, in which case, awesome. But even if you do feel fine fetching different sizes and otherwise playing fitting room attendant for your besties, keep in mind that turnabout is fair play. If your friends aren't willing to do the same for you while you try on jeans at Lane Bryant, it might be time to find other people with whom to plan mall outings.

It might also be time to finally "come out." We don't mean

about your sexuality, whatever it is. We mean about being fat. If you are shopping with your thin friends, and they head over to the latest super-trendy-and-cheap-clothes-that-are-meant-to-be-disposable clothing store without a thought, remind them that, hey, you can't actually shop there, because they don't carry anything that will fit you. It's possible that they didn't even realize that, or it just didn't occur to them.

If that's the case, your friends probably aren't being malicious. We're all really bad at judging what size people wear. Marianne once posted a full-body shot on the Rotund and invited people to guess her height and weight. The guesses varied by over six inches and two hundred pounds—demonstrating that people have no idea what any particular weight actually looks like. Unless you have explicitly told them, your friends probably have no idea what size you wear. And they might be more than willing to tag along with you to Lane Bryant or the Avenue or Torrid, if you let them know you need to go to those stores. (If they aren't, then reread the chapters about getting better friends.)

However, if playing fitting room attendant has grown old, and you usually leave the mall feeling like a sad sack of awful who doesn't deserve nice things, you might want to consider a boycott of stores that don't carry your size.

YOU DON'T NEED ANOTHER PAIR OF EARRINGS

Readers, we are going to tell it to you straight: You don't need to shop at stores that don't carry your size. Plus-size stores carry things that fit you (well, to a point—there's a definite dearth of options available at the mall for anyone over a size 26, though online retailers are increasingly filling that gap). Stores that carry your sizes also have plenty of cute accessories—accessories, we might add, that are designed to fit you: bracelets that will fit over a chubby hand, necklaces that hang at the proper length, and chokers that don't literally live up to the name.

Really, that's a win-win situation. And we all want more of that. So when you find yourself in a store with adorable stuff that doesn't come in plus-sizes, write to their corporate head-quarters and let them know why you won't be spending any money with them, even on their non-clothing items. The next time you're dragged into some trendy shop where the largest pair of pants wouldn't make it past your knees, don't just wait patiently for your friends while feigning interest in a tiny jew-elry display. Get the address for corporate headquarters and send them something like the following example letter.

Dear _____,

I'm writing to let you know that, unfortunately, I will not be spending any money at your store, even on non-clothing items. Your decision to stop at a size 14, even though half the women in America are a size 14 or larger, eliminates me as a consumer. I love your selec-tion of accessories, but I can't in good conscience spend money to support a company that doesn't value plus-size women as customers. My dollars will be spent at a retail space that is inclusive of women like me.

The letter itself may or may not have any effect, but writing it will, if nothing else, help reinforce your own belief that you're a valuable customer who deserves the same respect and options as a thin person. You might not convince them to cater to a broader market, but you don't have to take their neglect with a smile.

CHAPTER TWENTY

Don't Keep Clothes That Don't Fit

One oft-mentioned baby step toward body acceptance is ditching those clothes in your closet that do not fit you at the size you are now. It seems like such an obvious, smart idea when you hear it. But then you stand in front of your closet and actually start looking at your clothes. Maybe you can just keep this *one* thing because, hey, it fit two years ago, and it was expensive, and you just never know . . .

People always seem to want to argue with this one. And there are one or two reasons (such as pregnancy or predictable weight fluctuations) why keeping clothes that don't fit you right this minute might be okay. But, in the vast majority of cases, clothes that *do not* fit you are just going to make you feel bad and take up space that could be occupied by clothes that *do* fit you.

Imagine it: You're getting dressed, and you open your closet doors or dresser drawers and pull out item after item that does not fit you. (Wait, do you even have to imagine it? Or is that already what getting dressed is like for you?) Is there any way at all for that to be a positive experience? We don't think so. Having nothing to wear sucks, and too many women condemn themselves to that fate while waiting to magically lose weight so they can fit into some pair of jeans they "love" more than their own imperfect bodies.

Why punish yourself? Are you doing penance for your fat through your wardrobe? If you are, stop it. If you're reading this book, you have most likely spent years apologizing and atoning for the size of your body already, and where did it get you? You have better things to do with your time—like getting out and living, no matter what size you are.

CLEANING OUT THE CLOSET

Clothes that don't fit you take up more than just valuable closet real estate. They take up mental space, too. They speak out every time you look at them, and the things they say are not helpful. "Oh, you looked so good at a size 8. If you just ate less and exercised more, you could fit into me again." Where have we heard that logic before? Oh, right, from the multibillion-dollar diet industry that would have us believe all bodies ought to be essentially the same, no matter what one's age, physical ability, or life situation.

Screw that.

Stop making excuses. Clean out the closet. Box up everything that doesn't fit you. Stuff the box(es) in the attic, if you truly can't bear to part with those acid-washed jeans you used to wear in high school. Otherwise, find a donation center and pass those clothes on to people who will benefit from them a lot more than you currently do. If you don't have a local Goodwill or don't want to donate to them, check out organizations like Dress for Success or the Cinderella Project, charities that collect business-wear and prom dresses, respectively, for low-income women. (From what we hear, they are always in need of more plus-size clothes, so if your "skinny" clothes are above a size 14, more's the better.) Consider sending your clothes to one of the many NOLOSE clothing swaps or the Fat Girl Flea that happens each year—details of which you can find online.

If you have a lot of clothes and a lot of patience and want to recoup some of your investment, it's also possible to make money from your old clothes. Consignment shops and auction sites like eBay allow you to earn cash for new clothes but still send your beloved old ones to a good home—a home where they aren't relegated to the back of the closet or the bottom drawer.

The most common excuse we hear when we suggest this exercise to people is that they can't afford to buy a whole new wardrobe. But, really, if you aren't wearing these clothes, you already *need* a new wardrobe, whether you like it or not. A closet full of clothes that don't fit doesn't give you any more options than an empty one. And clothes that just sit there taunting you and making you miserable cost you a lot more than just money.

Sell your old clothes and reinvest the funds in some new wardrobe pieces. Learn to sew and make new stuff or scour the sale racks and invest in one piece at a time. You'll wind up, even if it takes a little while, with clothes that fit your body now—and that is worth a lot.

Depression Pants
On Buying Things Too Small as a Motivational Tactic

by Lesley Kinzel

For the past several years I've had the unenviable experience of being a crazy-obsessive shopper and clotheshorse, while also being a size right on the cusp between levels of fatness. Not the inbetween-misses-and-plus size that folks wearing a 14 or 16 or 18 struggle with; I haven't been there for any appreciable length of time since seventh grade. No, I refer to the size between plus and, um, plus-plus, as defined by the apparel world.

See, these days a great many more designers and manufacturers are producing plus sizes, and for this I am certainly grateful, as well as pleased to have more options for places to spend my money. But it seems a surprising number of them have chosen to stop at a 24. I can wear some 24s, in some items, but generally speaking, me and 24 are but passing acquaintances: You know, like that guy who lives in your building that you see in the elevator all the time, and you know he told you his name at some point, like a year ago, but you don't remember it, and now you've been exchanging friendly-but-terse hellos in the hall and by the mailboxes for so long that asking him to refresh your memory would just be unbearably awkward, so you just say "Hi" and leave a pause in there where his name would go if you remembered it, before quickly moving on to discuss the weather or his dog's intestinal disorder or . . . whatever.

Me and 24 are exactly like that.

I know where 24 lives, I can recognize 24 from a distance, and yes, I can even wear a 24 now and then, depending on the item, but 24 and I ain't tight by any definition. (Well, except literally.) These days, when this size-24 cutoff and I meet face-to-face—most often, it seems, with department store brands or higher-end designers—I am angry. Really, really angry. *"But I want a pony!"* irrational-type angry. Before I inspire a million exasperated sighs, I'm well aware that manufacturers can't make every size in the world. I am also aware that I am not a precious and unique snowflake. But I'm still angry, because I really wanted that dress/sweater/pair of tights/wide, tricked-out belt/ruffley pirate shirt, and on and on, and I am only thwarted by said designer/manufacturer's failure to make it in a size I can wear.

I used to get angry about this as a teenager, too, but the anger then wasn't directed at the offending party—it was directed at myself, my body. It was my stupid body's fault for not fitting whatever size happened to be on the rack. Stupid body! You should fit those random-size pants! You disgust and embarrass me, body!

All of this brings me back to the popular "motivational tactic" that inspired the above-noted ruminations in the first place: the practice of purposely buying clothes too small with the intention of dieting one's way into them. These are garments not simply too tight or uncomfortable, but garments intentionally purchased in a size too small to even get oneself into. I've known several people over my lifetime (all women in my case, though I'm sure this is a habit indulged in by folks of both genders) who've bought things—usually dresses—and kept them as Magical Talismans to drive them to weight loss, fitting into that size as much a measurable goal as attaining a certain number on the scale. A friend in high school had such a dress that hung, at all times, on her closet door. So she got to look at it every day; it was the first thing she saw when she woke up in the morning and the last thing she saw before falling asleep. It became this fetishistic little totem—the day that dress finally fit was the day Her Life Would Begin.

Is that the most depressing dress-related thing ever, or what?

I can almost understand this behavior, at least from the position that, yes, often I've wanted to wear a certain garment and been thwarted by the garment's not being available in my size. It's frustrating and infuriating for sure. But it's not my body's responsibility to fit into some frilly container, arbitrarily shaped by someone who doesn't even know me. It's not my body's fault a size 20 won't fit, it's the size 20's fault; let's think about that, shall we?

And let's think about how totally counterproductive and just plain weird it is to purchase something you can't even wear, for the purposes of driving yourself to fit what Insert-Retailer-Name-Here requires. Isn't that downright abusive of the body you've got, the body that likely got you to the mall in the first place, that moves you through the world? Is it kind or loving to parade some unfitting Dream Dress before that body, reinforcing its failure to be some randomly chosen size? Isn't that kind of hateful and unhealthy? Doesn't that body deserve better?

Part of this stems from my own selfish belief that nobody should put off looking fabulous. Buying a dress too small for the purposes of motivating (or guilting) oneself into smallening one's body enough to fit it is putting off fabulousness in a most heinous sense, as it assumes that your fatter body is not worth wearing something beautiful that fits and that you love. Because showing off implies self-acceptance and confidence, two things that, culturally, fat folks aren't supposed to have.

Fabulous is not size-dependent, it's confidence-dependent, and if you ain't confident in yourself at a size 26, it's unlikely that you'll be any more confident at a size 16 (or whatever your "confidence size" might be). Real, lasting self-confidence comes from feeling secure in the person you are, not what you look like at a given moment in time.

PART SIX

{ **The Media** }

CHAPTER TWENTY-ONE

Train Yourself to Read Media Reports on Fat and Dieting with a Critical Eye

When we were in college working toward our respective English degrees, we both frequently heard the mantra, "A liberal arts education teaches you how to think." (This is supposed to make you feel better about the fact that it does not teach you how to make money.) Kate recalls feeling rather put out by that statement when she first heard it—she already knew how to think, thank you very much!—but eventually, she realized that people actually meant, "learning how to think *critically*." As in, researching, questioning, looking up your sources' sources, checking your own biases, learning to spot others' biases, and making connections that might not be obvious on the surface. That's the stuff that eventually gets you a BA, if not a high-paying job. And it's the same stuff that will help you read media articles about THE OBESITY CRISIS BOOGA BOOGA BOOGA, without collapsing from either the weight of self-loathing or the terror of your imminent death by fat.

The media reports on a new study ostensibly proving something or other about fat, food, and/or exercise literally every day. But how often do you question the sources of this information? Who did the study you're reading about? Who funded it? How big was the sample size? What were the actual numbers? How was the study designed? Is there a difference between the conclusions the researchers published in a peer-reviewed journal and the take-away message you're hearing on the evening news?

For that matter, is there a difference between the researchers' data and their own published conclusions? Part of what sold us on the idea that all the obesity crisis hype is just that was reading books like Paul Campos's *The Obesity Myth* and J. Eric Oliver's *Fat Politics* (more on those in the next chapter), which looked at some of the very same studies that have led to so many articles about the dangers of fat, and found that the raw data simply does not warrant all the panic. By looking closely at and thinking critically about the information that was already out there, Campos and Oliver both found that the numbers had been manipulated to paint a falsely alarming picture. Digging deeper is always a good idea.

You don't have to be a scientist or a statistician to ask the important questions. (Campos and Oliver are both lawyers.) You just have to be curious about what's *not* being said in the articles you read about obesity research. Given that years long studies are often summed up with a few paragraphs of ink in a mainstream publication, you can be sure that you're almost never getting the whole picture, even if a given journalist has done her level best to be thorough and accurate. And what if she hasn't? Is the reporter truly objective? Do you see evidence of bias in the piece?

When you stop taking media reports at face value and start asking questions about the information they're conveying, you empower yourself as a consumer of information. Never forget that's what you are. Most media outlets are for-profit businesses; they're selling you something, and you decide what you're willing to buy, literally and figuratively. Once you start asking questions about what lies behind the articles you read or the newscasts you watch, you can begin to get a much better sense of where the truth lies and how easily it can be manipulated to push a particular agenda or to appear—ironically enough—more "consumer-friendly."

That advice to think critically goes for this book, too. We've included endnotes so you can check out for yourself where we're getting our info. We've only drawn on sources that we've deemed credible after a great deal of thinking and questioning. We've avoided sources that support what we're saying but have an agenda other than finding the truth. (For instance, there's one organization that puts out a lot of information on how the obesity crisis is overblown, much of which tracks with what we've come to understand and are relaying here. Unfortunately, that organization happens to be a front for the restaurant industry. Their purpose is to encourage people to spend money on eating out, not to promote well-being—much less truth for its own sake. So we'd never quote information from that source alone, even if we agree with it, because we can't trust that they're being intellectually honest.) We're a couple of bloggers with English degrees who happen to have done a lot of reading on this subject. It's up to you to question the quality of our information and our integrity in bringing it to you. This chapter will give you some tools for doing that.

FOLLOW THE MONEY

When you read about a new study that found fat is unhealthy in yet another way, do you ever ask yourself who paid for that study? Or who's paying the "expert" some reporter called for a response? Probably not—and sadly, neither do many of the journalists who write about such studies. For example, lots and lots of them regurgitate statistics or call on experts from the American Obesity Association. But a glance at the AOA's website[1] reveals that their sponsors include:

- Abbott Laboratories
- American Society for Metabolic and Bariatric Surgery
- American Society of Bariatric Physicians
- Amgen, Inc.
- Bristol Myers-Squibb
- Eli Lilly and Company
- Ethicon Endo-Surgery
- GlaxoSmithKline
- International Federation for the Surgery of Obesity
- Jenny Craig, Inc.
- Johnson & Johnson
- Knoll Pharmaceutical Company

- Medeva Pharmaceuticals

- Merck

- Novartis Nutrition
  Corporation

- Pfizer

- Regeneron

- Roche

- Sanofi-Aventis

- Slimfast

- Weight Watchers
  International, Inc.

All of those pharmaceutical companies, if you haven't guessed, are developing or already pushing weight-loss drugs. Kudos to the AOA for being transparent, at least. But here's an organization that has, according to their own website, "become an authoritative source for policy makers, media, professionals and patients on the obesity epidemic"—while their funding comes from commercial weight-loss programs, pharmaceutical companies, and doctors who stand to profit from performing risky surgery on fat people! Conflict of interest, anyone?

And don't assume the government-funded research you hear about is much better. In his 2007 book *Good Calories, Bad Calories: Challenging the Conventional Wisdom on Diet, Weight Control, and Disease*, Gary Taubes writes:

> Policy and the public belief are often set early in a scientific controversy, when the subject is most newsworthy. But that's when the evidence is by definition premature and the demand for clarification most urgent. As the evidence accumulates, it

may cease to support the hypothesis, but altering the conventional wisdom by then can be exceedingly difficult.[2]

Let us repeat that. *Altering the conventional wisdom by then can be exceedingly difficult.* Quick: Do you believe saccharine causes cancer? If you said yes, that's exactly what he's talking about (and the example he uses). If you said no, you're probably just too young to remember when the media was constantly telling us that drinking diet soda would lead to a slow, painful death— right before NutraSweet showed up to save us all. As Taubes points out, scientists concluded over twenty years ago that saccharine is not, in fact, harmful to your health—but all most of us remember is the panic that came on the heels of early studies that said it was. Because there was some inconclusive evidence that saccharine might be carcinogenic, there was a media blitz to get the message out before scientists were even sure if the message was true. When the early studies on a potential public health issue actually get it right, that kind of quick action is awesome—but too often, they don't, and we all end up freaking out about nothing.

Taubes goes on to point out that trying to promote a new public health initiative "requires unconditional belief in the promised benefits," even if the medical community hasn't quite achieved consensus on those benefits yet.

But if the underlying science is wrong—and that possibility is implied by the lack of true consensus—then this tendency of public-health authorities to rationalize away all contradictory evidence will make it that much harder to get the science right. Once these authorities insist that a consensus exists, they no longer have motivation to pursue further research.[3]

Or, more precisely, they no longer have motivation to pursue research that might undermine the authority of a gazillion existing government directives to eschew certain kinds of foods and always be vigilant about your weight. And what that means is, it's no longer in the government's best interest to fund studies that might leave them with egg—hey, remember how eggs were gonna kill us all, and then they weren't, by the way?—on their faces.

Now, we're not trying to get all tinfoil hat on you here. There's no big conspiracy. What we've described is shameful in scientific terms, but it's also human nature. We all want to believe what we want to believe, you know? If a bunch of rigorously designed, long-term studies come along and prove that, say, permanent weight loss really is possible for a significant percentage of people, we won't be thrilled about having to admit we were publicly, repeatedly wrong. But we will admit it, if it ever comes to that—and we're always curious about new research on fat and weight loss, whether it supports our preconceptions or not. That, apparently, is the difference between us and the U.S. government.

So basically, we've got a situation where there's loads of obesity research going on, but the vast majority of it is being backed either by private corporations that have a vested interest in promoting weight loss or a government that has a vested interest in supporting its existing claims about diet and health. Then we've got journalists reporting on the findings that come from that research without acknowledging potential conflicts of interest. (And often, it seems, without even reading more than the press release about a given study.)

MURDER AND ICE CREAM

That's just the beginning. Quick: How many deaths are associated with obesity in the United States in a given year? Did you say 400,000? That statistic—from the Centers for Disease Control and Prevention circa 2004—is still being bandied about in the media, even though it was revised down to 112,000 in 2005, after research led by Katherine Flegal, published in the *Journal of the American Medical Association*, showed the methodology of the previous study was seriously questionable.[4] There actually was a fair amount of buzz about the Flegal study and the CDC's official revision of the number, but plenty of journalists missed the memo. As we're writing, the most recent instance we've found of the "400,000" statistic in a reputable publication was in the July 2008 *Economist*. But whenever you're reading this, take a second to do a Google news search on "obesity 400,000"—we'll bet you a nickel you find at least one current example of your own.

"But wait," you're saying. "112,000 still sounds like an awful lot!" Sure, but that brings us to the cardinal rule of critical thinking: Correlation does not equal causation. There's an example often used in Sociology 101 classes to illustrate this point: In the summer months, both ice cream sales and murders increase, meaning there's a correlation between ice cream sales and murder. Now, in theory, once a correlation has been established, it's worth looking into whether one thing causes the other. Does ice cream trigger homicidal impulses? Do murderers like to celebrate a job well done with a nice waffle cone? No, probably not. In fact, heat is what causes the rise in both ice cream sales and homicide. Correlation does not equal causation.

So, yeah, there's an established correlation between obesity and excess mortality, but that doesn't tell us that being fat leads to early death. What it tells us is that something common to many obese people sometimes does lead to early death—and fat ain't the only thing a lot of fatties have in common. It could be lack of physical activity. It could be poor diet. It could be the stress of constantly getting ostracized and berated for being fat. It could be a history of weight cycling because we're so often told that one more diet will be the key to permanent thinness. All of those things are correlated both with increased mortality rates and with obesity. But most of the research that's done is so narrowly focused on proving that fat itself is the culprit, scientists rarely bother to separate out those other variables. Which means a fatty who exercises, eats her veggies, meditates, and never diets might not be in a high-risk category at all, but we'll never freakin' know, because everything is skewed so far in favor of blaming adiposity itself.

Pissed off yet? We're still not done. Quick: Are obesity rates on the rise? If you said yes, you're sure not alone in believing that—but you and everybody and their grandma are wrong. In 2007, the CDC released a report saying, "Obesity prevalence has not measurably increased in the past few years." Based on their National Health and Nutrition Examination Surveys, "there was no significant change in obesity prevalence between 2003–2004 and 2005–2006 for either men or women."[5] Furthermore, there had been no increase in obesity among American women since 1999! By the time you read this book, it will have been at least ten freakin' years since obesity rates leveled off for the ladies, but we're willing to bet the last time you heard an unqualified "Obesity is on the rise in America!" was more like ten minutes ago. Increasing obesity rates have become a "truth" so taken for granted, media outlets don't even bother to fact-check that shit anymore.

ON THE BIAS

Which brings us to bias. Not just the kind of bias that comes from being bankrolled by folks whose livelihood depends on the public believing we must lose weight to be healthy, but the more personal kind that often informs even ostensibly objective writing. You can randomly select any ten mainstream media articles on fatness in America, and we guarantee you'll find phrases like *packing on the pounds*, *ballooning*, and *thundering*— little bombs of editorializing in the standard science reportage. Each article will most likely be illustrated either with a photo of a headless fatty in a sweatsuit or a close-up of a forkful of cake going into a mouth residing just above a double chin. The headlines will all indicate that fatness is linked to something terrifying, no matter what the articles are actually about.

And even if a given article is—mirabile dictu—about how fat is not necessarily a looming public health catastrophe, it will usually end with a quote from an "expert" saying, "Yes, but . . ." As in, Yes, but people shouldn't take that as an excuse to sit around eating doughnuts all day. Yes, but there are still other studies that tell us fat kills. Yes, but I've built my professional reputation on demonizing fat, and I'm not about to give it up now. Okay, maybe not that last one. However, the "Yes, but . . ." sentence will almost always be there, right at the end. Don't get us wrong—we do understand that journalistic conventions require that "both sides of the story" be presented. But once you're aware of it, you'll be amazed by how often journalists give antiobesity crusaders the last word, even in the rare article suggesting that a big ass might not be a death sentence.

Journalists live in this culture just like the rest of us, which means most of them are very much predisposed to believe fat is dangerous, losing weight is "healthy" for all but the very thin, and fat people usually get that way by sitting on the couch scarfing bonbons. If those are your basic beliefs about fat, of course you're naturally going to cast a skeptical eye on the studies that challenge your assumptions and think much less critically about those that support them. The problem is, journalists are supposed to be trained to cast a skeptical eye on everything and keep their biases out of their work. But when it comes to reporting on fat, that doesn't often happen. From the headlines to the illustrations to the snide lines about "packing on the pounds," most reporting on fat reflects the work of multiple people who are quite obviously disgusted by it.

So if you're going to read mainstream media articles about fat, weight loss, or THE OBESITY CRISIS BOOGA BOOGA BOOGA—and frankly, unless someone's paying you to write about them, we recommend you just don't—you need to remember that what's there is (A) often distinctly colored by headline writers', photo editors', and reporters' negative opinions about fat, and (B) almost never the whole story.

Always look beyond the press release, even if actual journalists don't bother. Find out who funded the study in question. Try to read a copy of the study yourself, or even just the abstract—you'd be surprised how often the results, reported with due caution in a scientific journal, look a hell of a lot different from the sound bites that end up on TV or in newspaper articles. In fact, a lot of studies actually disprove the need for hysteria when it comes to obesity—not that the mainstream media is interested in covering that angle. Google the "experts" quoted to find out whom they represent and whether they have a history of anti-fat crusading. Basically, just use your brain. A little critical thinking combined with a little research will often reveal that the picture for fatties is not nearly as bleak as it seems.

CHAPTER TWENTY-TWO

Read Up on Fat Acceptance and the Science of Fat

Have you ever had a book really change your life? We're both the kind of voracious readers/nerds for whom that's happened several times, but still, there are books that stand out among the standouts. And there are few things that changed our lives quite as much as our respective shifts from typical self-loathing larger woman to Proud Fatty—for which books were largely responsible.

The beginnings of Marianne's self-acceptance came when she was a child watching daytime television. (Shut up.) There was a group of people talking about being self-respecting fatties and an audience full of people making fun of them. The memory of that show cropped back up when, in college, Marianne read Susan Bordo's *Unbearable Weight* and opened her eyes to the oppressiveness of our beauty ideals and the possibility of living happily in a fat body.

Not that, you know, she automatically started being happy

in her fat body at that point. After all, hating her body was such a comfortable thing to do—she was used to it, and rejecting all the dominant social thought about fatness was scary! But the idea of the beauty standard being used as a way to control women and their appetites (for food, for power, for sex, for whatever) was not so easily dismissed. Bordo's discussion of "the tyranny of slenderness" was not something she could just walk away from. And, despite more than a few subsequent rides on the dieting roller coaster and the self-loathing merry-go-round, Marianne eventually talked herself into giving *not* dieting a try.

For Kate, it was Paul Campos's 2004 book *The Obesity Myth* that really cemented the change in her thinking. *The Obesity Myth* made a whole lot of things fall into place in her mind all at once: that it is possible to be fat and healthy simultaneously; that diets really, really don't work; that so much of fat hatred is bound up in classism and racism. (Generally speaking, poor people are fatter than rich people, and African-Americans and Latinos are fatter than white people. Ever notice how much overlap there is among stereotypes of fat people, low-income people, and people of color? Do "lazy," "ignorant," "smelly," "dirty," and "stupid" ring any bells?) It made her grasp for the first time that being fat is neither a sin nor a death sentence, and that she'd be much better off if she focused on bolstering her physical and mental health, regardless of where her weight landed, instead of fighting the natural size and shape of her body. That's the power of a good book.

TAKE A LOOK, IT'S IN A BOOK

We're hoping, of course, that this book will be a life-changer for you—but we also want to encourage you to read widely about fat acceptance, body image, beauty standards, and Health At Every Size. For starters, we know this stuff can seem really out there when you first encounter it. *Wait, what? Fat isn't necessarily unhealthy or unattractive?* But the more you read, the more you realize the Fat Acceptance Movement (or Fat Liberation, Fat Rights, Body Acceptance, Size Acceptance—it goes by many different names, with different shades of meaning) isn't just a bunch of fringe types "looking for an excuse" to be fat, as our critics so often charge. (Who needs an excuse?)

It's a bunch of people—including medical doctors, nutritionists, psychologists, and a heck of a lot of smart cookies from various backgrounds—who have looked at the big picture and found that a fat-hating culture does serious psychological damage to so many, without actually eliciting the health benefits that are used to justify the hatred. It's a bunch of people who believe there must be a better way to promote good physical and mental health for fat people than shaming us and demanding that we diet again, again, again—for the rest of our lives, if necessary—or have risky surgery to become thin. And it's a bunch of people who are sick to death of hearing stereotypes and flat-out lies about fat people thrown around in the media, of seeing themselves or their fat loved ones discriminated against in employment and housing situations, of being the brunt of jokes, of being shown and sometimes told outright that fat folks are not worthy of the same respect and dignity accorded to other human beings. Reading lots of different books on the subject—whether by academics, science journalists, or plain-old pissed-off fat people—is a great way to get a feel for the many facets of the movement.

Books are also the best place to find well-drawn arguments against the specious science that's used to fuel fears of THE OBESITY CRISIS BOOGA BOOGA BOOGA. In addition to *The Obesity Myth*, we highly recommend J. Eric Oliver's *Fat Politics*, Gina Kolata's *Rethinking Thin*, Gard and Wright's *Obesity Epidemic: Science, Morality, and Ideology*, and Linda Bacon's *Health at Every Size* for their in-depth research into the facts about fat and dieting, which often don't match up to what's reported in the media.

THE FAT-O-SPHERE

In addition to the many books on the subject (see the appendix for more suggestions), in the last few years, the number of fat acceptance blogs has increased substantially. When we started blogging in 2007, Paul McAleer's Big Fat Blog—going strong since 2000—was almost the only game in town. Others had been started and abandoned, and still others were promoting body positivity as a general concept but also discussing weight loss alongside that. (We adore the ladies behind Big Fat Deal, but they aren't anti-dieting, and you might have noticed by now that we really, really are.) Some feminist and cultural criticism blogs were touching on fat acceptance, but it was never their primary focus. So into that not-quite-void came the Rotund and Shapely Prose—and then, before we knew it, dozens and dozens of others. We have no idea why 2007 was the Year of the Fat Blog, but some sort of Internet tipping point was achieved, and poof! The fat-o-sphere was born.

The great thing about the fat-o-sphere is that it's a smorgasbord of different takes on fat acceptance, body image, sexuality, disability, and self-esteem. Granted, most of the bloggers at this writing are both white and female—hardly a representative portrait of fat people in America or anywhere else—but as the fat-o-sphere grows, its authors are becoming more diverse in terms of nationality, ethnicity, socioeconomic status, gender, sexuality, and political leanings. We can't say there's something for everyone there, but there's something for a lot of different people—and hey, it's all free. If you're not ready to shell out for a book about fat acceptance (other than this one, obvy), all you have to do is check out the fat-o-sphere feed (see appendix). You'll find more than enough information there to keep you busy for a long time.

The best thing about the fat-o-sphere, though, is not necessarily the gold mine of fierce, funny, informative writing. It's the sense of community. Most of the blogs encourage readers to comment, and the discussions are sometimes better reading than the posts. (Yes, even on our blogs.) By and large, people are incredibly supportive of each other, which really helps to mitigate all the pressure we get from family, friends, and perfect strangers to feel ashamed of our bodies and try to become thinner. Lots of people (including us) have found real-life friends in the fat-o-sphere—and as we discussed earlier in the book, having a social circle that includes other women who aren't constantly talking about their diets or berating their own bodies is a major positive step toward self-acceptance. (Also, the commenters on our blogs have to be some of the wittiest people on the whole freakin' Internet.)

The very best reason to read books and blogs about fat acceptance and Health At Every Size, though, is to learn enough to come to your own conclusions. If this is the first you're hearing of it, we actually don't want you to simply take our word for it that the obesity panic is way overblown, it's possible to be fat and healthy, and you will not die alone if you never lose twenty (or two hundred) pounds. We want you to do your own research, examine your own feelings, and figure out what makes sense to you and what doesn't. We're pretty confident you'll eventually decide that hating your body doesn't make one darn bit of sense. But that can be a pretty major paradigm shift for a lot of people, and it doesn't always sink in right away. Reading as widely as you can is one of the very best ways to internalize the message that your body is not a problem to be solved.

CHAPTER TWENTY-THREE

Quit Watching So Much TV

True story: Several years ago, Kate quit watching TV entirely, just because she got busy with other things (*cough* Internet addiction *cough*). After about six months of no TV, she realized her body image was much better than ever, even though she hadn't been consciously trying to improve it. At first, she didn't put two and two together, but eventually it dawned on her that the only women she saw in a given day were average women in the real world—not actresses who are paid ungodly amounts of money to remain stick thin. And next to those average women in the real world, she didn't look so bad at all. Go figure! Likewise, Marianne hasn't even had cable since 1995. In addition to feeling better about her body, she has lots more spare time to spend writing and making things.

Ah, the television. The first regularly scheduled television broadcast began in 1925, and Americans haven't stopped watching television since. So, what's wrong with that? Is there really a problem with coming home after a long day (or flipping on the TV during the middle of the day) to sit down and relax in front of whatever the networks are offering us?

In theory, of course not! It's not like you are relaxing by kicking puppies or anything. But, in practice, if you are working hard to get the negative messages that our culture feeds us about fat bodies out of your head, sitting in front of the television is pretty much totally counterproductive.

THE BEAUTIFUL PEOPLE

Think of what you see in a typical hour of TV. Lots of very thin women, whose livelihoods depend on them remaining very thin (meaning it might make sense for them to spend hours a day at the gym, but that doesn't mean we all can) and who are attended to by a team of stylists and makeup artists before they ever step in front of the camera. Even if they're meant to look like they're wearing no makeup, they're wearing makeup, and even if they're playing schlubby characters, they're wearing clothes you probably can't afford. They don't have bad hair days, because trained professionals make sure of that. Their skin looks flawless. Their shoes are amazing. This is what's presented as "normal" for women on TV.

If you see a fat woman during that hour—and that's a big "if"—she'll be presented as either a joke or a bitch, and there will probably be a scene of her stuffing food in her face, regardless of where she is or what else she's doing—usually with crumbs trickling down her chin, as if she's baffled by the purpose of napkins. She will likely be seen throwing herself at a man who has no interest in her, with zero awareness of his feelings. She will have no clue that the other people around find her unattractive and pathetic. This is what's presented as "normal" for fat women on TV.

And every few minutes, those images will be interrupted by ads exhorting you to buy products that will make your hair shinier, your skin clearer, your teeth whiter, and of course, your body smaller. You can be just as beautiful as those "normal" women on TV, if only you're willing to lay out the money!

Seriously, you need to turn that shit off.

HIDE THE REMOTE

Some of you are going to be mad about this. You're going to say we're overreacting and that we just want to take your favorite show away from you. Well, we promise, we aren't out to get you—and if you continue to watch your stories, we aren't going to think less of you. (Kate's even gotten into a few new shows again after that enlightening total moratorium on TV, but she does highly recommend TiVoing or downloading your favorite shows, so at least you can skip the advertising.) Nevertheless, we're still going to tell you why the decision to stop watching television, or at least seriously reduce our TV consumption, was one of the best decisions either of us have ever made.

Think about the women you work with, the ones that you join for coffee, or that you see at any point when you go about your day. Now think about the women on TV. While we are (mostly) sure that they are lovely people, their bodies do not reflect the average body of your everyday woman. For that matter, no one on television (except for maybe the fat men who are constantly being portrayed as the bumbling husbands of modelesque wives) has a really average body. Do you remember when we told you to spend some time looking at a wide variety of bodies, especially fat bodies? Watching TV, with its homogenous portrayal of female beauty, doesn't really mesh with that. In fact, if your goal is to surround yourself with diverse images of women, watching TV is one of the worst things you can do.

We know, we know, logic is cold comfort when you really just want to veg out to some sitcom. We sympathize. And still, we suggest you leave the TV off for the most part—pick up a book or hang out on some blogs or Internet forums. Try it for a week. If you think you don't have time for the hobbies we mentioned in Chapter 11, you might be surprised at just how much free time you create. That is time that can be spent at a book club or a class, at the dog park, or out with friends at a wine tasting. Or, you know, playing video games (which can also be body image pitfalls, but Raving Rabbids is just too much fun).

While you're at it, even if you really love checking out the latest styles (which don't come in size fat anyway), lock your women's magazines away for a week, too. If you pore over the images presented in fashion spreads, you are going to internalize that image as the ideal. That's bad both from a fat/body/size acceptance perspective and from a feminist one. Women in fashion magazines are posed in highly passive positions and are almost always overly sexualized. These magazines are trying to tell you that if you just look and dress a certain way, you'll be irresistibly desirable. But you are more than an object. And, as we've discussed quite a lot, you are desirable just as you are anyway.

After a week of this media diet—the only kind of diet we recommend—check in with yourself. Do you have more free time? Are you spending even a little less time obsessing about your body's perceived imperfections? If yes, rock on. Keep it up for another week. If no, give it another week anyway. Your peace of mind is worth the experiment.

We're not trying to say that there is absolutely nothing of value on TV or in women's magazines. If you turn off the TV for a few weeks and discover that you're feeling bad about missing it more than about your body, at least you have a clearer head with which you can now watch your favorite shows—pay attention and see if the cultural messages still seem so harmless.

You might find yourself happy to watch a single show—maybe even one with a diverse cast and an interesting plot, that never resorts to cheap jokes at the expense of people who don't look like models. (Hey, we can dream.) Or you might find yourself switching it off and leaving the house to meet friends and go do something more fun. Something that doesn't make you think you're an ugly piece of crap who needs to lose fifty pounds and exfoliate more often.

PART SEVEN

{ Getting Your Head on Straight }

CHAPTER TWENTY-FOUR

Get Over Yourself! They Really, Really Aren't All Looking at You!

Marianne and her friend Mark made up a little song that they like to sing to each other sometimes, to remind themselves that most people are too self-absorbed to pay much attention to what other folks are doing. You can make up your own melody to go with the words:

> 99 percent of the things that people do
> have nothing to do with you.

(Note that it's important, no matter what melody you choose, to draw out that last note on "you.")

It might sound kind of harsh—but the truth is that most people are not walking around with you as the center of their universe. People are generally the center of their own universes. So when you are sitting on the subway, humiliated because you just realized your shirt is on inside out, chances are good that no one else has even noticed. (Hey, it took you that long to notice, and you're in the shirt!)

And those assholes who do notice? Their response isn't about you or your value as a human being. It is rooted in their own issues. Maybe they had a traumatic childhood experience involving an inside-out shirt, or maybe they were raised by their parents to think such a thing was at the top of the shameful things pyramid. Either way, that has nothing to do with you.

Now, you can't assume that everyone who calls you a name necessarily hates themselves, but you *can* remember that these people are being fed the same cultural messages as you are. They just may not have questioned those messages and examined the status quo the way you have. Which means—sing it with us—their issues about your appearance have nothing to do with yooooou.

STRANGERS AREN'T ALL THAT

We don't say this so that you can walk around feeling superior to those living the unexamined life. We just think it can help to understand that everyone, not just fat people, are getting the cultural message that fat is bad—and not everyone has thought about rejecting that. It's going to take a while for society at large to catch up—and in the meantime, you get to practice not caring what other people think.

That's what it comes down to, after all. Marianne is pretty sure that, to the average person walking down the sidewalk, she represents a hot mess of a person. Her hair goes everywhere, her clothes don't generally match (on purpose, but not everyone gets that), and oh yeah, she's fat. But that random person has no power over Marianne's life. Why should she choose her clothes to suit their tastes? Especially when bright colors and pom-pom trim make Marianne really happy?

Kate, likewise, favors clothes that do nothing to draw attention away from her fat, and she's even had "friends" say things like, "Isn't that print a little loud for, you know, someone like you?" (You know, a total fucking fatass?) No, as it happens, that print is only a little loud for someone who doesn't like loud prints. For someone like Kate, it's perfect.

Some people's opinions matter, of course. If Kate's boyfriend, Al, is embarrassed to be seen in public with her, that's something Kate will want to address. (She'd usually choose to address it with "Get the hell over it," but then, Al doesn't usually give a rat's patoot what she wears, so it works out fine for both of them.) If Ed can't take Marianne anywhere because he thinks she's coming off as a little too much, that becomes a problem for both of them. Kate might change her shirt (or she might not) and Marianne might quiet down (or suggest a different restaurant if the venue is really the problem). You make special allowances for the people that matter to you—either because the relationship has proven they might have a valid point or because you love them enough to sometimes work around their issues.

But why would you extend that to the skeevy dude at the end of the bar who has been pointing and laughing at you all night? Why should his opinion matter?

The easy answer is that his opinion *doesn't* matter, not in any real way. But in the real world, where you don't ever really get used to being mocked or ridiculed by the people you want to like you, it can be hard to fully believe that.

How do you do it? By figuring out what kind person you want to be, and what kind of style you want to have, for yourself—and working toward that. That means not depending on other people to show you who you are. If you're meeting your own standards of fabulousness every day, other people's standards don't matter so much.

It also means acknowledging that your mother was right: Other people aren't looking at you all of the time. They are too caught up in their own crap—and probably worried that everyone is looking at *them*. As more and more people accept themselves and work toward changing our culture, hopefully that won't be such a given. But even when that happens, people still won't be looking at you! They'll be too busy going about their own fabulous business.

Marianne finally figured out that, when she cared about what strangers thought of her body, it really came down to fear; she was afraid that no one would like her or find her attractive and—since she was buying into the cultural messages at the time—she didn't really even like herself or find herself attractive either. Blocking those cultural messages, and really working to like herself, made a huge chunk of that fear go away. Putting herself out there made it easier to find other people who did like her and who did find her attractive. But she wouldn't have met any of them if she hadn't decided that strangers weren't going to determine her self-image.

If there were an easy way to come to that conclusion, we'd probably be writing that book instead (or, at least, as well). But you are on the right track, reading this book right here. Learning to accept yourself on your own terms makes it a lot easier to dismiss the opinions of random skeevy dudes.

The Wages of Visibility

by Lesley Kinzel

To set the scene: I am fortunate enough to live, with my dear husband, in a condo on a fairly popular beach. During the summer, I go out to the beach quite often—even after work, on weekdays, since this time of year sunlight persists past 8 p.m. at my latitude. Some days I go with company, some days by myself. I don't so much go for tanning purposes (I'm heartily committed to SPF-a-million sunblock), but because I enjoy the beach, and the sunshine, and the ocean, and find my time there entirely relaxing and restorative.

Today, while waiting to cross the street to actually get on the beach, I got catcalled. By a slender white girl (teenaged, I would guess) riding in a big white SUV with an unknown number of other teenaged slender white girls. The car slowed down, and the sneering girl in the passenger seat yelled out the window at me, "Hey baby, can I hit that?"

In the hundredth of a second I had to respond, I did what came naturally, as if it were a remark leveled by a teasing friend. I smiled salaciously and called back with an exaggerated "Yeeeaaaah." And then I laughed. This elicited astonished looks and peals of nervous, brittle laughter from the occupants of the car, which then quickly sped away.

I knew, as I always know, that this couldn't have been intended as anything other than a sarcastic and just plain mean attack. It's been years—years!—since I've been catcalled like that, with unabashed malice as the motive behind it, so I was a little taken aback. I made my way onto the beach, down to where the quiet surf was beating the sand; I laid down on my towel and folded my arms under my head and thought.

It was gnawing at me.

I get angry when this shit gnaws at me.

I began my initial engagement with fat activism over ten years ago. Why the fuck can these experiences still gnaw at me? Why is it still possible for this to get under my skin, to unnerve me, to distract me from a beautiful afternoon on a beautiful beach? Who the hell do those people think they are, to feel entitled to fuck with my happiness, my choice to be out in public, to go about my life without being made to feel like a lesser being, like something that does not deserve these things? What do they gain by trying to ruin my day?

And then I thought: This is the wages of visibility.

This is what I get for being visible, for daring to go out, alone, dressed for the beach. This is what I get for refusing to hide, for refusing to apologize, for having the audacity to leave my house and live as though I've got nothing to be ashamed of. To a casual observer, it makes me a target. It makes me a fool. It makes me a pushover, an easy mark, a laugh. People will always want to remind me: You've got no right to be so happy with yourself. Fatty.

Catcalling sucks, no matter the circumstances. If it's sarcastic, it implies that no one could ever possibly find you attractive. If it's genuine, it implies that your body (and by extension, your sexuality) is public property and simply being outside is an open invitation for commentary. Either way, it's depersonalizing, and objectifying, and it sucks. I tend to think the long absence of the sarcastic catcall from my own life is likely rooted in my carriage and self-confidence; it's difficult to effectively tear down somebody who's obviously not feeling badly about herself, and I expect that my unhesitating reaction to the catcaller today was the reason for the astonished looks as the car drove away. I also think my built-in catcall-avoidance is at least partly a result of my age; women who aren't so young (I'm only in my 30s, but still) are seen, culturally speaking, as less sexual, less objectifiable, and thus their fatness is less an affront. For example, I doubt the girls in that car would have catcalled a woman their mother's age.

Given that ultimately catcalling is always a commentary on a person's attractiveness, either positive or negative, it tends to take place within a certain set of parameters. Though I was hardly thinking this deeply at the time, my reaction to the catcalling teenagers may have inadvertently addressed both their assumptions of my apparent sexual unattractiveness (vis-à-vis my fatness) *and* of my perceived straightness, by my instant response in the affirmative to a sexual advance made by a female, in spite of that advance's obvious insincerity.

There are so many people—people my size and far smaller—who wouldn't even consider going to the beach, or wearing a swimsuit in public, for this very reason—the fear that someone will look, someone will say something, that someone will make them an example, that they will be humiliated, that they will be made to feel like they've got no right to leave the house wearing anything less than a tent, looking the way they look. And that makes me angry, that we can let people dictate to us what we can do, and where we can go, out of fear of instant humiliation that could come at any time, humiliation that the perpetrator will likely forget within the hour, but which the embarrassed person may carry with her for days, or for months, or for the rest of her life.

Given the choice between restricting my movements and being assured of never being catcalled again, versus going out shamelessly and risking (or demanding!) attention—I will gladly take the latter. I like being visible. Even when I become a bull's-eye upon which the insecurities and savagery of others are exorcised. Even when I lose time processing and remembering the emotional risks I take just by being myself, time I would have otherwise spent relaxing in the sunshine. When I began my self-acceptance process, I decided first off that I never wanted to feel afraid of what those people—those who would mercilessly catcall me from a moving car, for example—might think or say about my body again. I never wanted to avoid life out of fear. And I'm still there, still fighting to be fearless.

So I say fuck those people. I'll be on that beach tomorrow, and this weekend, and for months to come, and if they don't like it, good, I'm glad to displease them.

They cannot stop me.

CHAPTER TWENTY-FIVE

Defend Your Own Honor as Vigorously as You Would a Friend's

Do you remember how we told you not to hang out with people who say negative things about your body (or their own bodies, for that matter)? Now ask yourself this: Based on those rules, how likely would you be to hang out with yourself?

You aren't going to let anyone call your best friend a fat, disgusting pig or tell her she doesn't deserve a relationship until she loses weight, right? You aren't going to take a plate of food away from her if she's still hungry or frog-march her to the gym and berate her until she finishes a workout she hates. Of course not. But we bet you've done all those things to yourself without even thinking about it.

This is where we tell you to knock that right off. You deserve to treat yourself just as well as you treat other people. You need to be your own best friend for a little while—and that doesn't mean ditching your actual best friend. In fact, you might want to recruit her or him to yell, "Stop hurting my friend!" every time you slam or deprive yourself. After listening to you hate on yourself for all those years, they might even find that cathartic.

ACTUALLY, IT ISN'T FUNNY

A lot of people, a lot of women in particular, use a sort of self-deprecating humor to put themselves down and make people laugh at the same time. It keeps us from looking arrogant (because confidence in women can be misread), and it plays into that gross way people bond over flaws (or diets). Look, you might think you are being witty and charmingly self-deprecating, but, really, you're not. Maybe you are trying to head insults off at the pass—negative commentary can have less of a sting when we turn it into a joke ourselves. But by anticipating negative commentary, you are actually getting into the habit of creating more opportunity for it to happen.

Kate had a huge revelation years ago when a friend of hers from college told her, "You know, it's really uncomfortable for other people when you put yourself down. You're usually funny about it, so we want to laugh, except we don't want to sound like we really think those things about you . . . So it's really hard to know how to respond." In a twisted way, Kate had actually believed she was making people more comfortable by acknowledging the elephant in the room—her being that elephant, of course. But when she thought about it, she realized her friend was completely right. The problem wasn't that everyone was thinking about her fat and politely declining to comment on it—the problem was that she assumed everyone, even her friends, were as disgusted by her fat body as she was. In reality, her friends—being real friends—had no desire whatsoever to talk about how "ugly" and "disgusting" Kate was. She was the one who kept bringing it up—not only keeping the size of her body at the forefront of other people's minds, but alienating them with her *behavior*, not her physical repulsiveness.

Maybe it just feels arrogant to actually like yourself. A positive body image can, for sure, seem like arrogance when it's so routine for women to put themselves down and deny themselves the spotlight. But seriously, let's flip this one around. How arrogant is it to assume that everyone's judging your looks—that you know what they're all thinking, even if they're not saying it? Acting like you're a freakin' mind reader strikes us as a lot more delusionally egotistical than saying, "Yeah, I'm comfortable with the size of my thighs."

Negative self-talk, as the self-help books call it, really is damaging, and it's a habit you need to break. Sure, we're all equally unique snowflakes, and an attitude of entitlement bugs the crap out of any reasonable person in no time flat. But come on. If someone pays you a compliment, and your response is to talk about how big this dress makes your ass look, you might have missed the week in kindergarten where they talked about manners. The proper response to a compliment is "thank you."

This is one of Marianne's pet peeves, probably because it took her so long to get it through her head just how important this was. "You look nice" would trigger an automatic response like, "Oh, thanks, I really need to do something with my hair, and I usually wear more makeup." The bit about the makeup has never been true, by the way—Marianne doesn't wear it all that often. So, people would offer compliments, and she would, in effect, argue with them about why they were wrong. Which not only demonstrated her own lack of self-acceptance but actually insulted the taste of the people trying to compliment her.

If you have a hard time accepting and truly believing compliments, just practice saying thank you. No matter what your internal monologue winds up being, the words that come out of your mouth need to be, "Thank you." Think of it as good manners, think of it as fake-it-til-you-make-it, walking the walk you talk, or whatever else it takes to convince yourself to accept a compliment.

WHEN IT'S OKAY TO HATE YOURSELF

Defending your own honor is going to be hard. Actually, all of this work toward self-acceptance is hard. We won't lie to you about that. (Or, really, about anything else—that's one of the bonuses of having no shame.) But consider how unhappy you have been in the past, waging a war on your body, as though it were a malicious enemy. And then consider how pissed off you'd be at anyone who treated your best friend like that.

Now, get that pissed off at yourself. This is the one case in which we're willing to endorse a little self-directed anger. If you're going to hate yourself, at least do it for the right reasons, people! Hate yourself for being so mean to a perfectly good person—you. Hate yourself for being so arrogant you assume you know exactly what other people are thinking about you.

Hate yourself for being rude to people who want to compliment you. Hate yourself for hating yourself—hatred's no good!

Then forgive yourself, and start defending yourself from anyone who tries to make you feel bad—including you—just the way you'd defend a friend.

CHAPTER TWENTY-SIX

Accept That Some Days
Will Be Better than Others

If we lived in a land of sunshine and roses and kittens and unicorns and rainbows, then we would all be able to follow the steps outlined in this book and be totally okay forever.

It's a damn shame that we don't live in that world. Instead, we still live in a world that tells us fat is unhealthy, unattractive, and unassailable evidence of moral turpitude.

Tuning out those messages takes a lot of work, and, this being an imperfect world, our efforts are not always rewarded with a constant internal equilibrium. Both Kate and Marianne still have days when they catch themselves thinking, "Ugh, I wish my thighs/gut/boobs were different," or "Damn, I wish I could shop at regular stores," or even, "Maybe if I just went to the gym a little more, I could . . ." Walking the walk of this body acceptance stuff is an ongoing, daily effort, even for us.

We don't even know if it is possible to reach a place where these thoughts and the insecurities that drive them don't show

up. Sometimes we let ourselves hope that eventually, girls growing up in Western societies won't start out with those insecurities, so they'll never have to deal with unlearning them. But
in the meantime, all we can do is stop those thoughts in their
tracks before they spiral out of control.

The bad news is, that work is a pain in the ass that might just
last a lifetime. The good news is, unlike with dieting, it feels
great to get back on this wagon after you fall off.

THE DOWNWARD SPIRAL—NOT JUST A GREAT ALBUM

Why is it important to stop the negative spiral in the first place?
Because it is the kind of spiral that only leads down. Some days
you may feel like you are standing still, but at least you are
holding your ground against the surge of cultural messages you
take in every day. On the bad days, though—the days when you
hate your fat ankles and wish your chin weren't so pudgy—you
lose a little bit of ground. Your forward momentum, the stuff
that's been propelling you along the self-acceptance continuum,
is reversed. And if you don't work to turn yourself around,
you'll wind up right back where you started—or worse. Not
only do you want to avoid feeling shitty about yourself again,
but you don't want to have wasted all that effort—especially
not after reading all the way through to this point in the book!
So how do you stop those negative thoughts?

The first thing you have to do is accept that you are going to
have good days and bad days. If you think every day from here

on out is going to be a nonstop self-acceptance party and then one day you're sabotaged by your own brain, it can be devastating. When you acknowledge ahead of time that there will always be occasional troubles, you position yourself to successfully deal with the days when you feel like you are made to fail. This means you get to enjoy the good days a lot more, too, because you aren't taking them for granted.

OWN YOUR BAD DAYS

The next step in dealing with bad days is to let yourself own those feelings. "Own your feelings" sounds very cheesy and self-helpy, but let us explain. Part of accepting your body is living in it—connecting with your body. Owning your feelings means living in your feelings and connecting to them. Since hating on your body is often a proxy for dealing with other problems, admitting that you feel lousy about yourself long enough to ask why that is can be helpful.

For example, Marianne, during the writing of this book (because she is perverse this way), started to feel worse and worse about herself. Rather than deny there was a problem, she talked about it with a few friends: She felt tired all the time and like she wasn't a good writer and like she just wasn't interesting in any way, shape, or form. The people she talked to listened, empathized, and encouraged her to figure out where these feelings were coming from. It took a little while, but she figured it out; it had been an eventful year or so, what with turning thirty, getting married, getting laid off, becoming a contractor, writing this book. . . . All of this stuff was kind of over-whelming, and she was worrying about disappointing herself and everyone she knew. Once she knew what was going on, she could address it.

Figuring out the source of her self-criticism didn't magi-cally make it go away. But it meant she could be kind to herself and set more realistic expectations. It meant she could accept that *someone* is probably always going to be disappointed in what she has to say—the world is like that—but that the people who matter are still going to love her. And she is still going to be okay with herself, because failure, when it comes, is an oppor-tunity to learn something new and try again.

Marianne is, obviously, an optimist.

But she is also able to honor her bad days by treating her-self better when the negative thoughts come to town. If you try to bottle up the feelings from your bad days, they're going to explode in your face. Worse yet, if you start to identify as Little Miss Accepts Herself and then have a nervous breakdown in a fitting room, you're right back to feeling like a big, fat failure—exactly the habit we want you to break.

Want to know a secret? Even for a long time after she started blogging about fat acceptance and Health At Every Size, Kate still couldn't bring herself to do one form of exercise she knew damn well she loved: swimming. Why? Because swimming requires that she don a bathing suit (at least at the gym). Though she'd grown accustomed to wearing yoga pants and tight tank tops in public, she still was not quite ready to bare her thighs—historically, her most despised body parts—anywhere but the locker room. (And even there, she tried to avoid it.) As we've said many times, body acceptance does not come easily or all at once—it's a process. A long, slow process.

By the time she started blogging, Kate had obviously made a lot of progress toward loving her body, or she wouldn't have been writing about it—but she and her thighs still had some serious issues to work out. The happy ending is, after about a year of blogging and being involved in a thriving online community of fat-positive people, she finally got to a point where the appeal of swimming outweighed the fear of baring her thighs, and she went to her first water aerobics class. Better still, by that time she'd met another local fat blogger, and they started going to water aerobics together. It's a blast.

Now, indulge us for a moment while we count up how many of the points in this book are involved in that little story. Get over yourself—nobody's looking at you? Check. Find a form of exercise you love? Check. Defend your own honor as vigorously as you would a friend's? Check. (If one of Kate's friends said, "I love swimming, but I'm too embarrassed to wear a bathing suit," Kate would go nuts on her!) Read fat-acceptance blogs, hang out with body-positive friends, get a hobby and do it with other people? Check, check, check. We're not just making this shit up, people—we're telling you what has worked for us and what continues to work for us.

As more-or-less authorities on fat acceptance and developing a positive body image, we can feel like huge hypocrites when we have bad days, so we're sometimes loath to admit it. But every time we do admit it on our blogs, the comments and emails pour in from readers saying they're so relieved to hear that we still struggle with these issues—they thought there was something wrong with them, because they just couldn't seem to love their bodies all the time, when we make it look so easy!

Trust us, the last thing we want is for people to shift from "I'm a failure because I'm not thin and gorgeous like Gisele Bundchen" to "I'm a failure because I'm not self-confident like Kate and Marianne." If you take away only one thing from this book, let it be this: Be kind to yourself. That means not bagging on yourself for being fat or bagging on yourself for still succumbing to deep-seated insecurities. We all have them, and we all have lousy days. All we can do is try to recognize the negative thoughts for the bullshit they are, before they have a chance to take hold.

CHAPTER TWENTY-SEVEN

Don't Put Things Off
Until You're Thin!

You know that inspirational magnet saying, "What would you do if you knew you could not fail?" Well, our inspirational magnet, if we had one, would ask this: "What would you do if you knew no one would reject you because you're fat?"

We know you've got a list of things in your head that you'd like to try, but not until you lose weight. In fact, we're pretty sure the only women in America who don't have that list are longtime fat-acceptance activists and very thin or athletic women. Remember those statistics on how many women hate their own bodies? Setting aside how unbelievably fucked up and sad those statistics are, they certainly suggest that the vast majority of women in English-speaking countries, at least, have given some thought to how much better their lives would be if they could just get thin.

Wait, actually, let's not set aside how unbelievably fucked up and sad those statistics are. Instead, let's compare them to a couple of the statistics that are repeated ad nauseam to invoke the dread fear of fat: According to the National Institutes of Health, 61.6 percent of American women are overweight or obese, whereas only 36.1 percent are considered to be at a "healthy" weight.[1] And of course these stats rely on the body mass index scale, which doesn't take into account gender, age, frame size, or the difference between muscle and fat. But even taking those assessments at face value, you can see there's significant overlap between women who are not remotely "overweight" by any rational standard and women who want to be thinner. That fact really deserves a moment of headshaking silence. Go ahead, we'll wait.

So, if you're like most women, you believe that losing some weight is a prerequisite for being happy and self-confident—which means you've probably got that list of things you'll feel too insecure to try until you're thin (whatever value of "thin" is required by your own head). Taking a vacation alone, wearing a bathing suit in public, putting a dating profile online, getting back into the workforce after you've had kids, signing up for salsa lessons, presenting a paper at a conference—any of those sound familiar?

But if you've read this far, you know that dieting won't make you permanently thin. You know that treating yourself kindly, doing exercise you love, and eating when you're hungry are far more likely to promote long-term good health than trying to get skinny. You know there are people out there who really, truly will find you attractive just as you are. You know the media hype about fat is way overblown. And you know that

when you're sure everyone's staring at your abundant hideous-
ness (or hideous abundance, as it were), you probably just need
to get the hell over yourself.

So here's the real test of all that new knowledge: Stop putting
things off until you're thin. Go down that list in your mind and
find something you can do right now, something you can sign
up for tomorrow, something you can save up for. Get started.
Live your own damned life.

THE "FAT IS FINE FOR *OTHER* PEOPLE" PHASE

Once you've really started believing in fat acceptance—as
opposed to thinking it sounds nice for other people, but you
still need to lose X pounds before you'll be acceptable—it can
be hard to remember how you thought about these issues
before (just as it can be hard to imagine what it would really
be like to accept your fat body before you've done it). Like
pretty much everyone does upon first finding out there's such
a thing as fat acceptance, Kate spent ages in the cognitive dissonance phase: It made perfect sense that THE OBESITY CRISIS
BOOGA BOOGA BOOGA hype was way overblown—and even
if it weren't, dieting doesn't work anyway—but she still wanted
to lose weight and still felt like she, personally, needed to get
down to at least a size 10 before she could really get started on
her fat-acceptance journey. (Insert eye-roll.) These days, she can
certainly remember that she felt that way, but it is a lot harder
to really recall what it felt like to believe those two contradictory things simultaneously.

That sort of cognitive dissonance gives rise to a particular kind of resistance that shows up every single time we dare to say on our blogs that dieting doesn't work. It's the kind that essentially amounts to "Don't you take my hope away!" Those of us who don't believe in dieting are frequently accused of demoralizing fat people, of sending a cruelly pessimistic message when we acknowledge the simple reality that most fat people cannot become permanently thin. We've never quite gotten our heads around that one, because the message we're sending is that you're actually allowed to love your fat body instead of hating it, and you can take steps to substantially improve your health without fighting a losing battle with your weight. We're pretty sure that message is both compassionate and optimistic, not to mention realistic. But there will always be people who hear it as, "We, Kate Harding and Marianne Kirby, are personally condemning you to a lifetime of fatness! There's no point in trying, fatty! You're doomed! Mwahahaha!"

And that response reminds Kate of what it was really like before she'd actually made peace with her body. And what it was really like was this: The Fantasy of Being Thin absolutely dominated her life—even after she'd gotten thin once, found herself just as depressive and scattered and frustrated as always, and then gained all the weight back because, you know, diets don't work. The reality of being thin didn't even sink in after all that, because the Fantasy of Being Thin was still far more familiar, still what she knew best. She'd spent years and years nurturing that fantasy, and only a couple years as an actual thin person. Reality didn't stand a chance.

THE FANTASY OF BEING THIN

One problem with exhortations to quit putting things off and live your life now is that they don't take into account magical thinking about thinness, which we suspect is really quite common. We know that for us, the Fantasy of Being Thin was not just about becoming small enough to be perceived as more acceptable. It was about becoming entirely different people—ones with far more courage, confidence, and luck than the fat versions of ourselves had. It was never just, "When I'm thin, I'll look good in a bathing suit"; it was, "When I'm thin, I will be the kind of person who struts down the beach in a bikini, making men weep."

See also:

- When I'm thin, I'll have no trouble finding a partner or reinvigorating my relationship.

- When I'm thin, I'll have the job I've always wanted.

- When I'm thin, I won't be depressed anymore.

- When I'm thin, I'll be an adventurous world traveler instead of being freaked out by any country where I don't speak the language and/or the plumbing is questionable.

- When I'm thin, I'll become really outdoorsy.

- When I'm thin, I'll be more extroverted and charismatic and thus have more friends than I know what to do with.

- Et cetera, et cetera, et cetera.

In light of that, it's a lot easier to understand why some people freak out when we say no, really, your chances of losing weight permanently are virtually nil, so you'd be better off focusing on feeling good and enjoying your life as a fat person. To someone fully wrapped up in the Fantasy of Being Thin, that doesn't just mean, "All the best evidence suggests you will be fat for the rest of your life, but that's really not a terrible thing." It means, "You will never be the person you want to be! All the evidence suggests you will never find a satisfying relationship or get a promotion or make more friends or feel confident trying new things!" So if that's what you hear when we say, "Diets don't work," then yeah, we can see how that would be a major bummer.

PERSONAL LIMITS

Overcoming the Fantasy of Being Thin might be the hardest part of making it all the way into fat-acceptance land. And that might be why Kate had pushed that part of the process out of her memory: It sucked. Because she didn't just have to accept the size of her thighs; she also had to accept who she is, rather than continuing to wait until she magically became the person she'd always imagined being. Ouch.

That is, of course, a pretty normal part of getting older. You start to realize that yeah, this actually is it, and although you can still try enough new things to keep anyone busy for two lifetimes, you're pretty much stuck with a basic context. There are skills, experiences, and material things you will almost cer-

tainly never have, period. It's a challenge for all of us to understand that accepting this fact of life does not necessarily mean
cutting off options or giving up dreams, but simply—as in the
proverbial story about the creation of Michelangelo's *David*—
chipping away all that is not you. For a fat person, this can be
even harder to accept, because so many sources encourage us to
believe that inside every one of us is "a thin person waiting to
get out"—and that thin person is *so much cooler.*

The reality is, Kate will never be the kind of person who
thinks roughing it in Tibet sounds like a hoot; give her a decent
hotel in London any day. She will probably never learn to water
ski well, or snow ski at all, or do a back handspring. She can be
outgoing and charismatic in small doses, but she will always
then need time to recharge her batteries with the dogs and
a good book. She might learn to speak one foreign language
fluently over the course of her life, but probably not five. She
will never publish a novel until she finishes writing one. Smart
money says she is never going to chuck city life to buy an alpaca
farm or start a new career as a river guide. And her chances of
marrying George Clooney are very, very slim. Most of these
things are also true for Marianne, especially the outdoorsy
thing.

None of that is because we're fat. It's because we're *us*.

But when we were invested in the Fantasy of Being Thin,
we really believed that changing this one "simple" (ha!) thing
would unlock a whole new identity—this totally fabulous, free-
spirited, try-anything-once kind of chick who was effortlessly a
magnet for interesting people and experiences. And of course,

being fat then becomes an excuse not to do much of anything, because if it wouldn't be the *real* you doing it, what would be the point?

For Kate, accepting her fat really wasn't the hard part. Accepting her personality—and her many limitations that have zero to do with her thighs—was. But oddly enough, once she started to do that, her life became about a zillion times more satisfying. She found the right guy, took up yoga, started taking her writing more seriously. She stopped apologizing for taking vacations in the United States and Canada instead of somewhere more exotic. And lo and behold, being Kate Harding got a lot more fun. The thin person inside her finally got out—it just turned out she was actually a fat person.

GIVING UP VERSUS SETTLING

Giving up dieting and accepting our bodies didn't just mean admitting we would never be thin; it meant admitting we would never be a million things we might have been. (Which, we're told, is a phenomenon sometimes known as "maturity.") We absolutely do not recommend settling—which is where the confusion about pessimism comes in—but we do recommend self-awareness and self-forgiveness. There's a big difference between saying you *can't* be anything other than what you are right now and you *don't have to* be anything other than what you are right now. You will probably never be permanently thin, unless you are already, but other than that, the sky's the limit. You can be anything or anyone you want to be, in theory.

The question is, who do you really want to be, and what are you going to do about it? (Okay, that's two questions.) The Fantasy of Being Thin is a convenient excuse for not asking yourself those questions sincerely—and that's exactly why it's dangerous. It keeps you from being not only who you are, but who you actually could be, if you worked with what you've got.

And that person trapped inside you really might be cooler than you are right now. She's just not thin.

Don't Diet Anyway. They Still Don't Work.

But . . . but . . . but . . . !

Oh, we can hear you now. "But I need to diet!" Oh, really? Why's that? "Because this fat-acceptance stuff is fine for everyone else but not for meeeeeeeeeeeeeee!"

Uh-huh. Go back and reread Chapter 1. Reread the whole book, if you have to. It can be a hard pill to swallow, but you are really not such a special snowflake that dieting is the right answer for you, even though nearly everyone who does it ends up just as fat or fatter. Giving up on dieting isn't giving up on yourself—it's giving up on hurting yourself, starving yourself, and blaming yourself for things you can't control. It's giving up on engaging in culturally approved self-harm. It's giving up on authoring your own failure.

It's also freeing up a lot of time and energy that you can spend doing other things. It's freeing up the mental energy you need to learn a new hobby. It's letting your body have the fuel it needs to do something physical. It's ceasing to undermine yourself, so that you can meet new people with confidence and make some new friends.

It's giving up on the Fantasy of Being Thin and trading it in for the Realistic Prospect of Being Happy with Who You Are. Which of those sounds better to you?

KATE'S ACKNOWLEDGMENTS

Marianne Kirby undertook this project with me when neither of us had any idea if we could actually sell it. Then Molly Lyons came along and did just that, plus a whole lot of first-time author hand-holding (times two). Enter Meg Leder, who went to bat for us as necessary, made us better writers, and offered yet more hand-holding. All of these women have earned my gratitude and admiration like I can't even tell you.

My co-bloggers, "Fillyjonk" and "Sweet Machine," have made Shapely Prose a gazillion times smarter and funnier than it ever was when it was just me, and more important, they've helped keep me (more or less) sane in the face of trolls, fat-haters, and life in general. The "Shapelings" have turned the blog into a thriving community full of wit, wisdom, and support—something so much bigger than just a repository of rants. This book wouldn't exist without Shapely Prose, and Shapely Prose would pretty much suck without Fillyjonk, Sweet Machine, and the amazing commentariat, so huge thanks to you all.

Al Iverson has been there for me in so many ways I can't even begin to articulate why I'm thankful to and for him. Let's just say that getting wasted enough to hit on him might be the smartest thing I've ever done.

MARIANNE'S ACKNOWLEDGMENTS

When I founded the Rotund, I had no idea I would soon be friends with an amazing woman named Kate Harding. If our friendship had been the only thing to grow out of the blog, it would have been worthwhile. Lucky me, other people started reading the blog, too. I wouldn't wake up excited to write every day if it weren't for the amazing people who share their comments and their lives with me there.

Molly Lyons got this project from the minute we sent it to her. Her enthusiasm and conviction made this a better book when it was still just a concept. We also lucked out when Meg Leder took us on as first-time authors; her patience and understanding have been invaluable.

Man, I have so much to thank Lesley Kinzel for that I don't even know where to start. So, I'll keep it basic. Thank you, Lesley, for being in our book. Thanks also to Julia, Cynara, Joy, and Barb for their words and the fierce integrity with which they live. You guys rock so hard.

My husband, Ed, uses the word *fat* without flinching, reminds me to eat, and makes me laugh every single day. There's no way I could ever say thank you enough; hopefully, this is something of a start.

Body-Positive Resources at the Library

We recommend all of the following books for their ability to further illuminate issues we've touched on in Lessons from the Fat-o-Sphere. Be warned, however, that not all of them are entirely (or in some cases, even mostly) fat-friendly; they're just all worth reading, if you want to know more.

Bordo, Susan. Unbearable Weight: Feminism, Western Culture, and the Body. Berkeley, CA: University of California Press, 2004.

Campos, Paul. The Obesity Myth: Why America's Obsession with Weight Is Hazardous to Your Health. New York: Gotham Books, 2004. (Note: This was reprinted in 2005 as The Diet Myth and is now out of print under both titles, though it's available as an e-book from Amazon.com as The Obesity Myth. It's worth buying a Kindle. Seriously.)

Frater, Lara. Fat Chicks Rule!: How to Survive in a Thin-Centric World. Brooklyn, NY: Gamble Guides, 2005.

Gaesser, Glenn A. Big Fat Lies: The Truth About Your Weight and Health. Carlsbad, CA: Gurze, 2002.

Garcia, Megan. Megayoga. New York: Dorling Kindersley, 2006.

Glassner, Barry. The Gospel of Food: Why We Should Stop Worrying and Enjoy What We Eat. New York: Harper Perennial, 2007.

Kolata, Gina. Rethinking Thin: The New Science of Weight Loss—and the Myths and Realities of Dieting. New York: Picador, 2008.

Kolata, Gina. *Ultimate Fitness: The Quest for Truth about Health and Exercise.* New York: Picador, 2004.

McClure, Wendy. *I'm Not the New Me.* New York: Riverhead, 2005.

Poulton, Terry. *No Fat Chicks: How Women Are Brainwashed to Hate Their Bodies and Spend Their Money.* Toronto: Key Porter, 1996.

Shanker, Wendy. *The Fat Girl's Guide to Life.* New York: Bloomsbury USA, 2004.

Taubes, Gary. *Good Calories, Bad Calories: Fats, Carbs, and the Controversial Science of Diet and Health.* New York: Anchor, 2008.

Wann, Marilyn. *FAT!SO?: Because You Don't Have to Apologize for Your Size.* Berkeley, CA: Ten Speed Press, 1999.

Body-Positive Resources Online

Big Fat Blog: www.bigfatblog.com

The Coalition of Fat Rights Activists: www.fatrights.org

The Council on Size and Weight Discrimination: www.cswd.org

The Fat Underground: www.eskimo.com/~largesse/Archives/FU/index
.html

Fatshionista: www.fatshionista.com

Fatshionista Livejournal community: http://fatshionista.livejournal.com

First, Do No Harm: www.fathealth.org

International Size Acceptance Association: www.size-acceptance.org

Joy Nash's Fat Rant Blog: www.fatrant.com

Kate Harding's Shapely Prose: www.kateharding.net

National Association to Advance Fat Acceptance: www.naafaonline.com

The Rotund (written by Marianne Kirby): www.therotund.com

Notes from the Fat-o-Sphere RSS Feed: http://feeds.feedburner.com/
FatFuNotesFromTheFatosphere

Plus-Size Clothing Stores

Alight

Alloy

August Max

B & Lu

Casual Plus

Catherine's

Cato's Plus

C.enne.V

Cherished Woman

Ebay

Eddie Bauer

Evans

Fashion Overdose

Goodwill (seriously, they
have a plus-size section
in most stores)

IGIGI

Jessica London

Junonia

Just My Size

Kiyonna

L. L. Bean

Land's End

Lane Bryant

Lee Lee's Valise, Brooklyn

Maximum Woman,
Toronto

Monif C

Old Navy

One Stop Plus

Re/Dress, New York

Roamans

Size Appeal

Svoboda

Talbot's Woman

Target

The Avenue

Torrid

Ulla Popken

Vive la Femme, Chicago

Voluptuous Vixen,
New Orleans

Woman Within

Zaftique

ENDNOTES

Chapter 1: Accept That Diets Don't Work
1. Traci Mann, et al. "Medicare's Search for Obesity Treatments: Diets Are Not the Answer," *American Psychologist* 62 (2007): 220–233.

Chapter 2: Practice Health At Every Size, Including Yours
1. Marcia Wood. "Health At Every Size: New Hope for Obese Americans?" *Agricultural Research* 54 (2006): 10–11.

Chapter 3: Find a Form of Exercise You Love
1. D. Neumark-Sztainer, et al. "Shared Risk and Protective Factors for Overweight and Disordered Eating in Adolescents," *American Journal of Preventative Medicine* 33 (2007): 359–369.
2. Peter Muennig, et al. "I Think Therefore I Am: Perceived Ideal Weight as a Determinant of Health," American Journal of Public Health 98 (2008): 501–506.
3. Xuemei Sui, et al. "Cardiorespiratory Fitness and Adiposity as Mortality Predictors in Older Adults," *Journal of the American Medical Association* 298 (2007): 2507–2516.

Chapter 5: If You Think You Might Be Suffering from Depression, Get Help
1. Susan C. Wooley and David M. Garner. "Obesity Treatment: The High Cost of False Hope," *Journal of the American Dietetic Association* 91 (1991): 1248–1251.

Chapter 6: Find Body-Positive Doctors and Go to Them

1. Kelly D. Brownell and Rebecca Puhl. "Stigma and Discrimination in Weight Management and Obesity," *Permanente Journal* 7 (2003): 21–23.
2. Nicholas Bakalar. "Disparities: Obesity and the Odds of a Kidney Transplant," *New York Times*, January 1, 2008.
3. Mike Jarvis. "Hip, Hip, Hurray!" *Gainsborough Standard*, June 28, 2007.
4. Kelly D. Brownell and Rebecca Puhl. "Stigma and Discrimination in Weight Management and Obesity," *Permanente Journal* 7 (2003): 21–23.

Chapter 10: Stop Judging Other Women

1. www.nationaleatingdisorders.org.
2. www.nedic.ca.
3. Molly Watson. "Poll Shows Women See Size 12 as Overweight," *Wales Online*, March 19, 2007. Available at www.walesonline.co.uk/news/wales-news/tm_headline=poll-shows-women-see-size-12-as-overweight&method=full&objectid=18825185&siteid=50082-name_page.html.

Chapter 16: Seek Out Images of Happy, Healthy, Hot Fat Women

1. A. Romero-Corral, et al. "Association of Bodyweight with Total Mortality and with Cardiovascular Events in Coronary Artery Disease: A Systematic Review of Cohort Studies," *Lancet* 368 (2006): 666–678.

Chapter 21: Train Yourself to Read Media Reports on Fat and Dieting with a Critical Eye

1. www.obesity.org/AOA.
2. Gary Taubes. *Good Calories, Bad Calories: Challenging the Conventional Wisdom on Diet, Weight Control, and Disease*, page 70. New York: Knopf, 2007.
3. Ibid.
4. K. M. Flegal, et al. "Excess Deaths Associated with Underweight, Overweight, and Obesity," *Journal of the American Medical Association* 293 (2005): 1861–1867.
5. Cynthia L. Ogden, et al. "Obesity Among Adults in the United States—

No Statistically Significant Change Since 2003–2004," NCHS Data Brief Number 1, Hyattsville, MD: National Center for Health Statistics. 2007. Available at www.cdc.gov/nchs/pressroom/07newsreleases/obesity.htm.

Chapter 27: Don't Put Things Off Until You're Thin!
1. http://win.niddk.nih.gov/statistics/#preval

INDEX

activity level, 67
actual weight, 24
Adams-Gellar, Paige, 142–43
Adipositivity Project, 130
Agricultural Research, 14–15
alienation, through behavior, 204
Allan, Anjelica, 53
allergies, 20
all-or-nothing attitude, 65–66
American Journal of Preventive Medicine, 24
American Obesity Association (AOA), 170–71
anger, caused by catcalls, 198–201
anorexia, 27
antidepressants, 44–45
anti-diet, 14, 182, 216
   online, 125
   See also intuitive eating
anti-fat messages, 77
anti-obesity, 177
AOA. *See* American Obesity Association
appearance, others' reaction to, 193–94, 198–201
art
   culture and, 131–32
   voluptuous figure in, 129–30
asthma, 20
attraction, 83
   attitude and, 104–5
   to bodies outside mainstream ideal, 102
   self-hatred and, 105

Bacon, Linda, 182
beauty, fat women and, 103
beauty ideals, oppression and, 179–80
Beauty Myth Kool-Aid, 83
beauty standards, 4, 181
   controlling women, 180
BED. *See* Binge Eating Disorder
before and after photos, 6
Benesch-Granberg, Barbara, 58–63
Big Fat Blog, 182
Binge Eating Disorder (BED), 39
bipolar, type II, 45
birth of fat-o-sphere, 183
black communities, fat acceptance in, 96
blame, clothes vs. body, 141–43, 163–64
blind dates, 80–81
blog(s)
   body acceptance, 124
   cultivating friendship, 183–84
   fat acceptance in, 182–84
   fat community, growing, 183–84
   online support, 212
blood pressure, 10, 15
   checking numbers for, 72
   diastolic, 11
   family history, 73
   systolic, 11
blood sugar, checking numbers for, 72
BMI. *See* body mass index

body
    comfort with own, 129–31
    finding clothes to fit, 135
    making peace with own, 87–88, 216
body acceptance, 4, 77, 220
    accepting reality and, 218–19
    in blog, 124
    clothes and, 141–43, 158
    daily effort in, 207
    slow process of, 211
    See also Fat Acceptance Movement
body dysmorphia, 119
body image
    bad days, dealing with, 211–12
    clothes and, 141–43, 163–64
    culture and, 65
    depression and, 46–47
    develop positive, 211
    mental health and, 44–45
    normal representations, 128–29
    outside mainstream ideal, 102
    perceived, 120
    positive, maintaining, 204
    reading about, 181
    real, 120
    relationships based on, 78–79
    TV and, 188
    variations in, 128
    women and, 213
    See also self-image
body mass index (BMI), 53, 214
books, finding influential, 179–82
Bordo, Susan, 179–80
Botero, Fernando, 130
breakfast, 33
"Brick House" (Commodores), 96
Brownell, Kelly, 50, 51, 53

Campos, Paul, 168, 180, 182
Canadian National Eating Disorder
    Information Center, surveys on
    desiring thin, 88
cardiovascular disease, 10

catcalls, 198–201
causation
    correlation vs., 175
    of deaths, 175
CDC. See Centers for Disease Control and
    Prevention
Centers for Disease Control and
    Prevention (CDC), 174–76
checklist to progress of self-acceptance,
    211
cholesterol, 15
    checking numbers for, 72
    lipoprotein, 11
Cinderella Project, donating to, 160
classism, 180
Clooney, George, 219
clothes
    alterations, cost of, 138
    altering, 137–38
    body acceptance and, 158
    cost-per-wear, 145
    custom made, 136–37
    donating, 159–61
    fitting, 135, 144
    fitting to body, 140, 141–43
    handmade, 139
    importance of stylish, 144–45
    as inanimate objects, 135–36
    margins of error, 137
    as motivational tactic, 162–64
    as problem, 137, 140, 163
    recycled, 147
    selling old, 160
    shopping for, 140
    sizing, 142, 148–49
    thrift stores, 147–53
    women's sizes in, 136
commentary, implied, 118
    negativity in, 203
Commodores, 96
community
    blogging, 183–84
    engaging with, 100

exposure to real people in, 131
fact acceptance in black, 96
fat-o-sphere, 182–83
    online, 183
    online support and, 131, 211
    sense of, 183
compliments, accepting, 204–5
consumer indulgence, 153
conventional beauty, love beyond, 86
corporate headquarters, contacting,
        156–57
cravings, food, 33–34
critical thinking, 167–69, 178
    applied to research, 168
    in journalism, 177
    mortality rates and, 175–76
    rule of thumb, 174–75
    ulterior motives and, 169
culture
    art and, 131–32
    being fit and, 65
    a healthy person and, image of, 17
    image of "normal" weight, 127–28
    invisibility in, 14
    messages in, 194, 196
    pop, 97
    self-confidence and, 164
    weight loss and, 13, 24
    women and, 88–89
Curves, weigh-ins, 70

dating, online
    dealing with rejection, 84
    posting pictures, 82
    self-representation, honest, 83
dating, with help of friends, 80–81
deep vein thrombosis (DVT), 59
demand eating. See intuitive eating
depression, 16, 43
    antidepressants and, 44–45
    body image and, 46–47
    changing weight and, 47–48
    indicators of, 46

situational, 44
symptoms of, 44
weight loss to defeat, 47
diabetes, 11, 17
Diagnostic and Statistical Manual of Mental
        Disorders (4th edition), 44–45
dieting, 214
    all-or-nothing attitude, 65–66
    bonds over, 122–23, 203
    as crisis situation, 122
    excuses, 5
    giving up, 220, 222
    vs. HAES, 14–15
    Harding-Kirby Lifetime Diet Plan,
        28, 31
    health and, 15–16, 73
    health issues associated with, 11
    as hobbies, 99
    ineffectiveness of, 47–48, 222
    long-term, 5
    long-term studies of, 9
    media reports on, reading, 167–78
    negative health impacts, 73
    questioning research, 174
    short-term studies, 10
    statistics of long-term, 7
    weight loss and, 34
    yo-yo, 10–11
    See also specific diet programs
diets
    vs. HAES, 14–15
    vs. lifestyle changes, 7
    vs. time, 8
diet soda myth, 172
diet talk, 122–26
    on MySpace, 125
    at office, 124–26
    over dinner, 124–25
    substitute conversations, 123
discrimination, weight-based, 181–82
    by doctors, 50
    on streets, 199–200
    in treatment, 57

doctors
    avoiding, 59–61
    fat hatred and, 58–63
    fear and, 50
    finding fat-friendly, 54–56
    high standards of treatment from, 56
    prejudice by, 51–52
    researching, 55
    risky surgery and, 171
    stereotypes believed by, 50–51
    trusting, 56
    weight and, 49–50
    weight-based discrimination by, 50
doctor visits, 53–54
    emotional trauma and, 51–52,
        58–63
    weigh-ins, 74
Dress for Success, donating to, 160
DuBois, W.E.B., 92
DVT. See deep vein thrombosis

eating disorders, 24, 126
    behavior and, 16
    See also specific disorders
eating local, intuitive eating and, 38
eating regular, 33
Economist, 174
economy, thriving from insecurities, 86
Edison, Laurie Toby, 130
education, liberal arts, 167
elective surgery, 52–53
emotional habits, breaking, 209–11
emotional risks, taking, 200–201
emotional trauma
    doctor visits and, 51–52
    scale producing, 70–71
emotions, owning, 209–10, 216
ethical eating, intuitive eating and, 38
exercise(s)
    all-or-nothing attitude, 65–66
    as atonement, 23–24
    benefits of, 13
    forms of, 25–26

    for fun, 21–22, 24, 25–26, 64–65,
        67–68
    getting back to, 68–69
    guilt/regularity of, 64
    intuitive, 66
    leisure-time, 67
    as means of losing weight, 22–23
    outside of gym, 67
    pain and, 23, 67–68
    with work, 67
    See also workouts
expectations, setting realistic, 210
external experience, 22

family
    commentary, setting boundaries,
        116
    intuitive eating and, 36–37
    negativity in, 115
    self-appreciation around, 118
    standing up to, 115–16
Fantasy of Being Thin, 78, 216
    as excuse, 221
    giving up the, 223
    new identity crisis and, 219
    overcoming, 218–19
    stalling life, 217
fashion industry, history of, 136–37
fashion, ready-to-wear, 136
fat acceptance, 77, 179, 211, 218, 222
    activists, 213
    believing in, 215
    blogs, 182
    in black communities, 96
    blogs, history in, 182–84
    racism and, 93–97
    reading about, 181, 184
    TV as counterproductive to, 186
Fat Acceptance Movement, 181
fat admirers, 103, 104
fat and fit, 25
fat bias, 176–78
fat, blaming, 218–19

Fat Club, first rules of, 79–80
Fat Girl Flea, 160
fat hatred, 58–63, 181
Fat Liberation. *See* Fat Acceptance
        Movement
fat-o-sphere
    community, 182–83
    diversity of representatives in, 183–84
    friendship within, growing, 183–84
Fat Politics (Oliver), 168, 182
fat-positive communities online, 131
fat-positive images, 129–31
    resources for, 131–32
fat prejudice, in health care, 50–53
Fat Rights. *See* Fat Acceptance Movement
Fatshionista.com, 131, 140, 145, 147,
        151, 162
Fat Thrift Challenge, 149
fear
    of being unattractive, 196
    overcoming, 211
feeders, 102–3
feminism, 188–89
fetishists, 102–3
fibromyalgia, 17
figure(s), voluptuous
    in art, 129–30
    in photography, 130
financial supporters
    of Health studies, 170
    of obesity research, 173
    research and, 173–74
First, Do No Harm: Real Stories of Fat
        Prejudice in Health Care, 51–52
fit model, 136–37
    agency, 141
    measurements of, 142
    responsibilities of, 142
Flegal, Katherine, 174
food(s)
    benefits of nutritious, 13
    craving, 33–34
    forbidden, 31

good vs. bad, 30, 39
    neutral, 29–31
food intake, restrictions on, 7
forgiveness, 220
friend(s)
    be your own best, 202
    commentary, setting boundaries on,
        116
    dating help from, 80–81
    giving up, 114
    making new, 100, 115
    negativity in, 120
    nonjudgmental, 139–40
    self-acceptance and, 121
    self-loathing, 118
    shopping with thinner, 154–55
    thrift shopping with, 149–51
friendship(s)
    formed by blogging, 183–84
    mutual support in, 112
    superficial bonds, 122–23
friends, negative, 149–50, 195
    avoiding, 111–12
    dealing with, 111–14, 120–21
    mental health and, 114–15
    setting example for, 119–21
    shopping with, 139–40
    weight input, 111–13
Full Body Project, 130

Gard, Michael, 182
Garner, D. M., 47
Geissler, Cynara, 147–53
general practitioner (GP), 54
genetic predisposition to fatness, 17
glycemic control, 10
*Good Calories, Bad Calories: Challenging the
        Conventional Wisdom on Diet, Weight
        Control, and Disease* (Taubes),
        171–73
GP. *See* general practitioner
Great Migration, 92
guilt, irregularity of exercise and, 64

HAES. *See* Health At Every Size
Hamilton, Anthony, 96
happiness, 223
    perceived, prerequisite to, 214
    thinness and, 47–48
Harding-Kirby Lifetime Diet Plan, 28, 31
health
    all-or-nothing attitude, 65–66
    cultural image of, 17
    dieting and, 11, 15–16
    fat, 184
    fat vs. thin, 127–28
    HAES and, 16
    honoring, 216
    judging, 72
    negative effects of dieting, 73
    questioning research, 174
    scale and, 72
    weight as irrelevant to, 72, 176
Health at Every Size (Bacon), 182
Health At Every Size (HAES), 14, 55, 72
    anti-diet, 14
    approach to wellness, 54
    vs. diets, 14–15
    elements of, 16–17
    health and, overall, 16
    individual needs and, 17–18
    reading about, 181, 184
health care
    for fat people, 53
    fat prejudice in, 50–53
health issues
    dieting, associated with, 11
    focusing on appropriate, 73
    genetic components, considering, 73
health studies, financial supporters of,
        170
hobbies
    benefits of, 99–100
    dieting and self-loathing as, 99
    finding new, 98
    friends and, making new, 115
    time for, 222–23

honor, defending, 202
Horne, Lena, 95
humor, self-deprecating, 203
hunger
    lack of, 32–33
    as signal to body, 18, 23

IBS. *See* irritable bowel syndrome
illness, weight as reason for, 52–53
Implicit Associations Test, 51
injury, weight as reason for, 52–53
insecurity
    economy selling, 86
    overcoming, 207–8
    succumbing to, 212
intuitive eating, 16–17, 27, 28–29, 66
    adapting to moral restrictions and, 38
    desserts and, 123
    difficulties of, 40
    explanation of, 29–30
    family and, 36–37
    incorporating restricted budgets,
        35–36
    teaching kids, 37
    unclear signs, having, 32
    weight loss and, 34–35
irritable bowel syndrome (IBS), 17

jogging, 21
joint replacement, 52–53
Jones, Substantia, 130
journalistic conventions, 177
Journal of the American Dietetic Association, 47
Journal of the American Medical Association, 174
judgment
    fear of, 90
    as harmful to self, 90–91
    of others, 89–90
    reflecting back to self, 88
    standards, 88–89
    standards, impossible, 88
    subjective, 72
    women, of other, 87

Kinzel, Lesley, 162–64, 198–201
Kolata, Gina, 182

language, nonconfrontational, 124
    applying, 114, 116
leisure-time exercises, 67
lifestyle
    accusations of unhealthy, 13–14
    active, 66
lifestyle changes, 5, 6
    vs. diets, 7
    long-term, 15–16
Lincolnshire Primary Care Trust, 53
literature
    review of weight loss, 8
    weight-loss program's, 6
LiveJournal.com, 131, 147
living in present, 217
love, 85
    beyond conventional beauty, 86
    finding, 107

McAleer, Paul, 182
McDaniel, Hattie, 96
Mae, Olivia, 151, 153
mammies, 94
Mann, Traci, 8
maturity, 220
media
    altering ideal body, 129
    articles fatness in America, 176
    awareness of manipulations in, 169
    consumption of, 129
    demonizing fat, 176–77
    feminism and, 188–89
    on image and singles, 78
    negative messages in, 121
    obesity statistics in, 174
    objectivity of reporters in, 168–69
    reading reports on dieting, 167–78
    twisting reality, 178
    weight loss and, 24
media diet, 187–89

medical board, filing complaints with,
        56–57
mental energy, 222
mental health, 17–18, 43, 116, 180
    body image and, 44–45
    cleaning closet and, 159–60
    fat-hatred and, 181
    negativity and, 111–15
    shopping and, 154
    verbally abusive friends and, 114–15
meta-analysis of scientific literature on
        dieting, 2007, 8–10
Metz, Stephanie, 131
Michelangelo, 219
Mode, 131
models, 128
    Photoshop, 89
    See also fit model
Mo'Nique, 96
mood disorders, statistics of, 43
mortality rates, critical thinking and,
        175–76
motivational tactic, 162–64
myocardial infarction, 10–11
MySpace, 125

name-calling, 198–201
Nash, Joy, 141–43
National Eating Disorders Association, 39
    surveys on desiring thin, 88
National Health and Nutrition
        Examination Surveys, 176
National Health Information Center, 39
National Institute of Mental Health, 43
National Institutes of Health, 214
negative body talk, 111–13
negative self-talk, 204
negative thoughts, 208
negativity
    in commentary, 203
    contagious, 120
    dealing with, 111–15
    in family, 115

negativity (cont.)
  in friends, 118, 120
  metal health and, 111–15
  reversed, 208
Nimoy, Leonard, 130
NOLOSE clothing swaps, 160
NutraSweet, 172

obesity, 11
  attitudes toward, 50–51
  mortality, increasing, 175
  nurses and, 51
  rates, change in national, 175–76
  statistics in media, 174
The Obesity Epidemic: Science, Morality, and
      Ideology (Gard and Wright), 182
The Obesity Myth (Campos), 168, 180, 182
obesity research, financial supporters
      of, 173
OB-GYN. See obstetrics-gynecology
obstetrics-gynecology (OB-GYN), 54
Oliver, Eric J., 168, 182
online
  anti-diet, 125
  blog support, 212
  community, 183
  community support, 131, 211
  dealing with rejection, 84
  fat positive communities, 131
  posting pictures, 82
  self-representation, 83
  shopping, 146
online dating. See Dating, online
opinions, outside, 194–96
osteoarthritis, 10

Paige Premium Denim, 142–43
partners
  attracting more potential, 107
  confidence in, 104
  good vs. bad, 79–80
  long-term, 107
  standards for, 85

partners, finding, 77–79
  loving yourself and, 78
  See also relationship(s)
partner types
  compromising, 106–7
  preferential, 106
PCOS. See polycystic ovarian syndrome
Permanente Journal, 50
personality
  accepting, 220
  thin, 220–21
pharmaceutical companies as sponsors
      to research, 170–71
photography
  before and after, 6
  voluptuous figures in, 130
Photoshop and perfection, 89
physical activity. See Exercise(s)
plus-size clothing market, 135–46,
      155–56
polycystic ovarian syndrome (PCOS), 52
pop culture shaping stereotypes, 97
PostSecret.com, 108
public health authorities, 172–73
Puhl, Rebecca, 50, 51, 53

Queen Latifah, 96

race and societal expectations, 92
racial stereotypes, 93, 180
  fat acceptance and, 93–97
racial uplift, 92–93, 94
reading
  critically, 167
  for entertainment, 189
  to internalize self-acceptance, 184
  power of, 180–81
  reasons to, 184
  to understand fat acceptance
      movement, 182
reality, accepting, 219–20,
      223
rejection, dealing with, 84

relationship(s)
    based on image, 78–79
    See also partners
research
    critical thinking applied to, 168
    financial supporters, 173–74
    government funded, 170–71
    inconclusive scientific evidence,
        172–73
    motivation to pursue, 173
    obesity and increased mortality rates,
        175–76
    questing sources, 168, 174
    on weight loss, 173
resources, for fat-positive images,
    131–32
restaurant conversations, 124–25
retailers, plus-size, 131
Rethinking Thin (Kolata), 182
The Rotund, 155, 183
Rubenesque, 129–30
Rubens, Peter Paul, 129–30
runner's high, 19–20

Salvation Army, 152
scale
    digital, 72
    emotional trauma from, 70–71
    as judgment, 70
    power of, 71
    See also weight
scale, numbers on
    getting emotional, 70
    obsession with, 72
    relevancy to health, 72
science of fat, 179
scientific literature, on weight-loss
      programs, 8–10
self-acceptance, 164, 179, 223
    bad days, dealing with, 208–9
    checklist to progress, 211
    friends and, 118, 121
    as process, 201

reversed negativity, 208
    working toward, 205
self-appreciation around family, 116
self-awareness, 220
self-centered humans, 193–94
self-confidence, 82, 196, 214, 223
    culture and, 164
    independent of weight loss, 99–101
    judgment harmful to, 90–91
    maintaining, 194–95
    outsiders influencing, 193–97
self-criticism, identifying source of, 210
self-deprecating, 203
self-deprivation, 29
self-esteem, 108
    catcalls and, 198–201
    women's magazines and, 129
self-hatred
    attractiveness and, 105
    right reasons for, 205–6
self-image
    strangers and, 194–97
    TV and, 185
self-loathing, 123
    as hobby, 99
    impact on others, 119
    transition from, 179
self-representation, and online dating,
    83
self-respect, 179, 203, 205–6
self-talk, negative, 204
sewing
    machine, 139
    from patterns, 139
sexual fulfillment, 103
Shapely Prose, 183
shopping
    for accessories, 156
    mental health and, 154
    as motivational tactic, 162–64
    with nonjudgmental friends, 139–40
    online, 146
    plus-size, 162

shopping (*cont.*)
    plus-size stores, 155–56
    resources, 131
    scarcity in fat-o-sphere, 148
    with thinner friends, 154–55
    thrifty, 147–53
single, being, 77–78
    enjoying, 81–82
    media's answers to, 78
"Sista Big Bones" (Anthony Hamilton),
    96
situational depression, 44
size acceptance. *See* Fat Acceptance
    Movement
Skorch, 131
societal expectations, 92
socioeconomic boundaries, 36
Starkey, Julia, 92–97
stereotype(s), 180
    breakers, 93
    doctors, believed by, 50–51
    fat people, 21
    mammies, 94
    pop culture shaping, 97
    racial, 93
strangers
    dealing with, 201
    disregarding opinion of, 194–95
    as powerless, 196–97
    relationship to, 193–95
    self-centeredness in, 193–95
stress, 17
stroke, 11
style, individual, 195
swimming suits, overcoming, 200–201

Taubes, Gary, 171–73
television
    body-hating messages and, 98
    body image and, 188
    fat acceptance, as counterproductive
        to, 186
    history of, 185–86

how to quit, 187–88, 189
    self-image and, 185
    selling an image, 187
    women and, 186
thin
    being, 127
    fat vs., 127–28
    happiness and being, 47–48
    personality in fat body, 220–21
    wanting to be, 88–89
thinness and happiness, 47–48
thrift stores, 147
    negotiating pricing, 151–52
    plus-size sections, 148
    shopping tips, 147–53
time vs. diets, 8
transplants, 52–53
trapeze dress, 140
Tummy Tamer, 78
TV. *See* television

UCLA. *See* University of California
    Los Angeles
Unbearable Weight (Bordo), 179–80
University of California–Davis, 14
University of California–Los Angeles
    (UCLA) researchers, 8–10
uplift, 94
USDA Agricultural Research Service, 14

vegetarians and intuitive eating, 38
visible, being, 200–201
volunteer(ing) as hobby, 99–100

weigh-ins, 70–71
    doctor visits, 74
weight
    actual, 24
    average among American women, 127
    culture and "normal," 127–28
    depression and fluctuating, 47–48
    doctors and, 49–50
    excess, 24

injury and, 52–53
natural fluctuations, 73–74
perceived ideal, 24
as reason for illness, 52–53
statistics of American women,
214
See also scale
weight cycling, 10–11
weight loss
accomplishments beyond,
99–101
body positivity and,
182
consuming to encourage,
163–64
culture and, 13, 24
depression, to defeat, 47
dieting and, 34
drugs, 171
exercising and, 22–23
health and, 176
intuitive eating and, 34–35
life goals connected to, 217–18
media and culture for, 24
permanent, 7
research on, 173
weight-loss programs
funding from, 171
success rates of, 54
weight range, natural, 34

Weight Watchers, 5, 52, 60
ads, 4
food scale, 61
weigh-ins, 71
women
average size of American, 127
beauty and, 103
body image, 213
bonding topics among, 122–23
clothing sizes, 136
culture and, 88–89
fighting unreachable image of, 129
finding real, 128–29
judging other, 87
obesity among, 176
oppression of beauty ideals on,
179–80
self-esteem and, 129
social value of, 65
TV and, 186
weight statistics, 214
Women en Large project, 130
women's magazines, and self-esteem, 129
Wood, Marcia, 14–15
Wooley, S. C., 47
workouts, 20–22
Wright, Jan, 182

yoga as exercise, 21
yo-yo dieting. *See* weight cycling

Barbara Benesch-Granberg: Barbara lives in Madison, Wisconsin, with her husband and twin sons. She enjoys knitting, learning, and engaging in amateur media analysis. Barb dreams of the day when she will have time to give First, Do No Harm (fathealth.wordpress.com) and her own blog (thornacious.wordpress .com) the attention they deserve. She thinks of her mom often.

Cynara Geissler, Fatshionista.com: Cynara is a size twentysomething twentysomething writer/editor/arts administrator who's fat in (and at) the Canadian prairies. She contributes to Fatshionista.com and co-moderates the Fatshionista community on LiveJournal.com. She's committed to size acceptance, HAES, thrifting, wardrobe remixing, poetry, and D, her partner of the last seven years (though not necessarily in that order).

Lesley Kinzel, Fatshionista.com: Lesley blogs at (and is the admin behind) Fatshionista.com; she also co-moderates the Fatshionista community on LiveJournal.com and has more than a decade of engagement with fat activism. For a living, Lesley works in higher education administration and has two graduate degrees. Having escaped her hometown in south Florida at the tender age of eighteen, she currently resides in the Boston area with her husband and their two demanding cats. Her hobbies include photography, vegetarian cooking, being the Catalog Whisperer, playing Rock Band, and subverting the dominant culture via a cunning mixture of activism and fabulous dresses.

Joy Nash, FatRant.com: Joy is an actress, writer, and fit model from Los Angeles. Her YouTube videos have garnered more than 1.5 million views and have been honored to be among the most-discussed online videos of all time. Joy's first video, "A Fat Rant," was recognized as an official honoree for the 2008 Webby Awards in the category of public service and activism. Joy has been featured on CNN, *Entertainment Tonight*, and in *Bust* magazine. A graduate of USC's School of Theatre and the British American Dramatic Academy, she's just finished a feature film with Michael Madsen and a sketch comedy pilot called "Fruit&Fly." Joy likes lumberjacks, crossword puzzles, and telling people what she thinks. Visit her website at www.joynash.net.

Julia Starkey, Fatshionista.com: Julia is a fabulous, fat, mixed-race, queer woman who lives in Cambridge, Massachusetts. Julia brings her love of intersectionality to the organizations she is involved with. These include groups that deal with fat acceptance, gender diversity, racism, sexism, and sci-fi. She earned a degree in folklore and mythology from Harvard University and is in the process of becoming a professional librarian. In her spare time, she sews herself fabulous dresses and bemoans the lack of patterns available for fat bodies.

Kate Harding is the founder of Shapely Prose (kateharding.net), one of the most popular blogs in the fat-o-sphere. A graduate of the MFA program in writing at Vermont College, she lives in Chicago and is at work on about seven different book ideas.

Marianne Kirby is the voice behind the popular fat acceptance blog the Rotund (therotund.com). A writer and artist, she lives fat and happy in Orlando, Florida, the land of year-round produce.